THE VETERINARY SUCCESS FORMULA

10 SOLUTIONS TO RUN YOUR PRACTICE SO IT DOESN'T RUN YOUR LIFE

SUSIE HIRSCH, DVM

Copyright © 2017 by SusieHirsch.com, Inc.

Find out how to make your practice into your dream practice and live the lifestyle you deserve at:

www.vetclinicsuccesssecrets.com

Introduction

This book was finally written because I wanted to help other veterinarians who are struggling with making their practices profitable, sane and fun places to work. I was in your shoes once. I'd like to share with you my story, so you know where I'm coming from.

Like many of you, I bought in to a successful practice after being an associate for a couple of years after graduation. That practice wasn't our idea of a perfect practice when my husband and I bought it in 1999, but it was profitable. Over the space of a few years we changed some things and had it just as we wanted, clients who loved us *and* their pets, and would do whatever we thought was best. We were in a big city, so there were lots of people and pets, and the economy was booming in those years. We even had the problem of being busier than we wanted to be. We started firing our pain-in-the-neck clients, charging new clients a non-refundable fee just to reserve a space in our schedule, and I cut my hours back to spend time with our kids. It seemed we could do no wrong. Then the lead ball dropped, literally, right in the middle of our clinic and our life. The city informed us we were in the way of progress, and they were going to take our practice by imminent domain to build a light rail system.

So, less than a year later, our practice and our livelihood was leveled. It was a big blow, both financially and mentally. What they had given us for the land ("fair market value" for real estate only, nothing for the business) wouldn't buy an empty lot in our neighborhood. So we thought long and hard and decided to move, head back to my roots, and headed to a rural area where no big city progress would touch us again. We thought the quality of life would be better, and it would be a better place to raise a family. The trouble was, we didn't know what a world of difference we were in for.

In the couple years of closing the old practice and opening the new, the economy changed. Things weren't booming like they had been. In fact, as you all know, it was one of the worst "recessions" in recent history! The location we moved to was a relatively poor county to start with, and most of the jobs were in mining and agriculture. And here people seemed to think of their animals differently, not so much as members of the family, but as workers with a finite value attached to them. We were stumped for awhile and our business didn't thrive like we had anticipated. In fact, it was hemorrhaging money! We had a building, equipment, a staff (how good they were is debatable) ... but so few clients and appointments each day. It was painful to look at the schedule in the morning. We had to use our credit cards to the limit and cash out my husband's IRA just to pay the bills and payroll!

Personally, we really had to learn to get by on the bare minimum. We were definitely not used to that! It was quite a shock, and the stress took its toll on our marriage, our kids, and our work. We had to sit down and have a serious conversation, actually, multiple serious conversations. Were we willing to keep doing this, putting our family through this stress trying to make this new business work? Would we be better off to declare bankruptcy and leave? We could always find work somewhere as an associate, we were both very good vets. Trying as the situation was, and as miserable as we were, we just couldn't give up. What can I say, we are stubborn, like I think most vets are.

So we had to find help. I went looking for it. I didn't really know what exactly I was looking for, but I was searching. We ended up hiring a business coach and participating in a year-long business growth group, and going more in debt. The program wasn't bad, but we were the first vets they had had in the group, and they weren't quite sure what to recommend specifically for our business. But I did learn a few things. I knew there was more out there, my perspective was definitely widened, and I just had to figure out how to get us to where we wanted to be and which part of what we learned we could use to get there.

We thought we were doing better and getting a handle on our business. We knew we needed to have a certain number of clients coming through the door each month, had a goal for the number of new clients in that total, and were SLOWLY getting more people in and up to almost breaking even financially. I could cover the most important bills and payroll. Then we had a month that just about killed us. We took a family vacation, the only one of the entire year, and returned to an absolutely dead clinic. What the relief vet brought in money-wise wouldn't even cover half her bill, let alone payroll. Appointments were trickling in, not the flood we expected upon our return. What was wrong with this place? What was wrong with us? We were panicked and at the verge of calling it quits, again.

I started searching for help again, in the middle of the night because I couldn't sleep for worrying about paying the bills. And then I came across a couple of resources that literally changed our lives and our business. I won't lie to you, over the course of the next few months we spent well over $50,000 dollars getting more information and learning how to apply it in our business and our life. But now we finally had the tools we needed, the knowledge to thrive in this economy, in this location, really in any location or economy. I thought we had been in business in two extremes- great economy, wealthy clients, valued pets, and bad economy, blue collar and middle class clientele, and 'just a dog' or 'just a cat' mentality. But really it was a matter of finding those keys that make a business work in any situation, in any economy.

I know that very few of you live in my extremes, and are much more likely just trying to improve your practice to make it a little busier, a little more profitable, a little less stressful. And that is great! Good for you. I'm glad you aren't going through what I went through. I wouldn't wish that on anyone. But these keys make a business work better no matter what or where. And they can make your life easier, less stressful and more fun. After all, didn't we get into this business because we love animals? Don't we get to go to work each day just to play with puppies and kitties? Maybe lambs, kids and calves, too? Ha. ha. That is what everyone else seems to think, isn't it? No wonder our burnout and suicide rates as a profession are so high.

But veterinary clinic life doesn't have to be like that, it doesn't have to look like that. Our practice now is a good place for me to go. I enjoy my staff and clients again (and there *are* clients to enjoy!). I don't dread payroll every other week, and stress about which vendors get paid each month. It has grown from a brand-new start up with 0 clients, to over half a million dollar practice in three years. In a small town of about 3000 people, in a rural agricultural area, in what qualifies as one of the poorest counties in Colorado.

These are techniques you can use in *any* clinic, *any* market and *any* economy. I have felt the pain, I have been there, and now I want to help other practice owners to get out of it, or avoid it entirely. Like I said, your situation probably isn't as extreme as mine was, and that is even better. You'll be starting from a better place than I did.

Why Should You Read This Book?

This book will help you unleash your talents (other than veterinary medicine) and your potential, by helping you navigate the business side of veterinary practice with ease and confidence.

This book will let you see what needs to be done in your practice to have a flood of new and existing clients coming in the door, have the staff in place to handle them when they do, and the easy steps you can put in place to make this whole process a system. One that runs whether you are there or not.

Isn't that what we all really want? The ability to have our practice run smoothly and profitably so we can concentrate on what we really love? For some of you that may be veterinary medicine. For others it may be managing the business side. And for some of you it might be panning for gold in Alaska! Whatever your greatest desire might be, you can make it happen.

You just need a little help fine tuning the systems that will allow your clinic to run smoothly, and find the right people to help you do that.

There is no reason you can't take time off and travel like your "human doctor" MD counterparts. After all, aren't we smarter than they are? Who doesn't know that it is harder to get into vet school than medical school? And now is your chance to take your practice by the horns (or the whiskers, as the case may be) and drive it where *you* want to go.

Acknowledgements:

I want to take a moment to thank my family. My husband Jeff puts up with all my forays into the dark world of business and marketing, while working the lions share at the clinic. He helps direct my energy and supports me in everything. I also want to thank our children, who lovingly participate in this crazy life, and bring more joy to me than I will ever be able to show them.

I also want to thank the coaches and mentors I've had during my career that have helped me get to where I am today.

And I definitely would not be here without the support of my clients, many of whom have become my friends over the years. All the animals I have treated and loved have honed my skills and compassion, and taught me so much.

Table of Contents

INTRODUCTION — 2

WHY SHOULD YOU READ THIS BOOK? — 7

ACKNOWLEDGEMENTS: — 8
Table of Contents — 9

CHAPTER 1. MAKE IT FUN! — 12
Office Humor - Need Some — 12
How Do I Make It Fun? — 12
Main Idea — 15

CHAPTER 2. EMPLOYEES — 16
Once Upon A Time — 16
The Down and Dirty — 16
Put It To Work — 22

CHAPTER 3. HATS & STATS — 24
Where Do I Belong? — 24
The Job — 24

The Bottom Line	30

CHAPTER 4. MARKETING BASICS   32

But Why?	32
The Down & Dirty Basics	33
Take Action	38

CHAPTER 5. KEEP IN TOUCH   40

Be Memorable	40
The Power of Showing Up	41
The Why and How	46

CHAPTER 6. PROMOTIONS   47

The Happy Client	47
What to Plan?	47
Top of Mind	52

CHAPTER 7. ALL ABOUT CLIENTS   54

Your Lifeblood	54
The Good Stuff	54
In Action	60

CHAPTER 8. CUSTOMER SERVICE RULES 62

The Game 62

The Plan 62

The Result 69

CHAPTER 9. THE HUDDLE 71

Why Meet, Don't We All Work Here? 71

The Schedule 71

Got It 77

CHAPTER 10. BUSINESS AS USUAL/COMMUNICATION 78

The Office 78

Put It All Together 78

The Long Haul 86

ABOUT THE AUTHOR 87

OTHER OFFERINGS FROM SUSIE 88

One Last Thing... 89

Chapter 1. Make It Fun!

"To succeed in life, you need three things: a wishbone, a backbone and a funny bone." - Reba McEntire

Office Humor - Need Some

Do you remember some of those long nights in vet school, everyone was exhausted after clinics, studying for boards, and just couldn't stop laughing? The power of fun, friendship, and laughter can transform something really grueling and hard into the stuff of fond memories. Where did the fun go? Sometimes it's hard to remember during long days, when nothing seems to go right, and you have much more to do than time to do it, that we got here because we actually *like* veterinary medicine. Owning a business can make you feel this way. But it doesn't have to. Bring some joy back into your job.

How Do I Make It Fun?

So, when you were a little kid, didn't you think that when you grew up you'd have a job that was fun? One that you loved, one that you had passion for? That's what this is *supposed* to be. That's why we all went to vet school. That, and we thought we could make a living doing it, too, which is another key component. But we all wanted to do something that we enjoyed. Something that we could do for our whole life, and like doing, not dread doing every day.

I know some people are slaves to their job. They wake up, they dread it. They hate going to work. They spend all day there, away from their family, come home, too tired to do anything, wake up the next day and do it all over again. And that's how they spend 40 years of their lives! That's not what I want. I assume, since you are reading this book, that's not what you want. That's not why we all went to school.

If that describes you now, and how you feel about your job, or the practice that you own, or the practice where you work, this book is going to help you have fun again. Get back to the point where you enjoy going to work, where you like what you do. You like the people you work with. And you *want* to go every day. And even if you don't have to work every day, and if you only *want* to work three days a week, you can! I'm going to show you how you can do that. How you can get that spark back, living your passion, doing what you went to school for, what you wanted to do with your life making a difference and making your life better as well.

How can we make work fun, even if you don't even enjoy going anymore? To answer this question, in order to make work fun you have to be the leader of the practice and determine the direction it will go. You have to be the one that sets the tone. You have to come in happy, bright, perky. Some days that's going to be a lie. Some days you're going to be putting on a face to act like that, but that's okay. This is your show. You have to set the example.

Another part of it is having the right people in place. You need people that enjoy their job, are good at what they do, and get rewarded for doing that. No one wants to come to work and do a good job and never hear an ounce of praise or get any financial reward for that. Having the right people in place is key to enjoying work and setting the stage for your whole team to enjoy it as well.

The bottom line is people want to be recognized in life. They want to make a difference. That's really what everyone wants. You have to give them the opportunity to do that, so you need to hire people based on their attitude and based on their past experience too. You need to know where they're coming from in life. You don't want someone that's always looking for something to complain about. You want someone who's always looking for how they can help, how they can do those things that are going to make a difference, that are going to get them recognized. They have to have that desire. That's kind of a core detail in their personality, really. This is something we'll address later in the chapter on employees, but this is where personality testing, as well as a great interview style, can really help you out when you're searching for the right people.

There are quite a few components that go into making work fun. When you show up to a well-oiled machine, and fit right in, that is an amazing feat. And that is fun! Having clients that you enjoy, being in an environment you like, and having your day scheduled the way you prefer all help combine to make work someplace you want to be. There are games that that make each day a challenge. Games that you can play with the staff centered around work. Even games that can include the clients. I'll give you some examples of things that you can do to get your clients involved. You can do this on social media. You can do it in the office. I'll go over a couple of those at the end of the chapter. So much of this comes back to the employees. You really have to have the right team in place to make your office run smoothly enough that you're willing to take the chance and have fun.

The truth is, a lot of us have been misled or almost conditioned not to have fun because we're always having to reprimand. We're always having to make sure things go well, and correct mistakes, and that isn't fun. Like I said at the beginning, you have to be the leader. You do have to lead by example and by attitude, but a lot of these framework pieces that we're going to be going over in this book are going to contribute to make it fun.

My goal is by the end of this book, going through the other nine chapters you're going to have the base work, the specs in place to make it fun. I debated about putting this chapter at the end of the book, but I also wanted to put it at the beginning to give you an idea of what you can expect and what life can be like at your clinic if you do these things, if you implement them, and if you're really committed to having the practice of your dreams. One that will run with you or without you because you have this great team and these great systems in place that are always generating new leads for clients, new clients coming in the door, and all the backend stuff is covered. Nobody's wondering, "Who should be doing this?" and, "It's not my job. Where is it going to get done?" You're not going to be wondering that either. Everyone is going to know where their place is, what their responsibilities are, and they're going to be wanting to do that. They're going to enjoy it or they're not going to be there.

MAIN IDEA

In conclusion, things are fun when you're winning, when you have a winning team, when you have a winning practice, when you have winning clients, winning cases. You're not going to win all the cases. We know that, but all those other things, they combine to make it fun for you, make it fun for your staff. Somewhere that you all enjoy being, and that's going to show. Your clients are going to see that. They're going to appreciate that. They're going to want to be a part of that.

Visit www.vetclinicsuccesssecrets.com **to get more ideas on how to get your practice to where you want it.**

Chapter 2. Employees

"Leadership is not about a title or a designation. It's about impact, influence and inspiration. Impact involves getting results, influence is about spreading the passion you have for your work, and you have to inspire teammates and customers." - Robin S. Sharma

Once Upon A Time

Have you ever had one of those days, where you try to do everything you can to avoid asking a certain person for help? Or feel like you are walking on eggshells around others? You know you're not the only one that feels it, too. Even the clients would tell you, if you asked, that there was something under the surface going on. Work, and more specifically, your clinic, should not be like this. It should be a place where everyone is there to help, to do their job, and advance the mission and goals of the hospital. If you've had those days, and are over the drama, you need this chapter to get clarity on how to work *with* your employees.

The Down and Dirty

Employees... I could write about this subject for hours! It's *so* important to what you do. Number one, to help you do your job better. Number two, to keep your clients happy. Number three, to make the practice run smoothly. Your biggest challenge is to get the right people in the right positions. I know that what we all say is our biggest headache and what we hate about owning a business is managing employees, but it truly doesn't have to be that way. I used to think that too. I don't anymore. That is probably my greatest joy or second greatest joy to happy clients.

Most of you are probably starting out with employees, you have a team of employees right now. Maybe they're the right ones, maybe they drive you crazy, maybe they're the wrong ones. Maybe they just need a different position. I don't know where you're at or where they're at but we'll get to where you want to be. First let's focus on getting new employees and than we'll address the current employees.

The key to getting the right new employees is having the right kind of hiring process in place. When you put an ad in the paper, or online, or wherever you advertise, you need an ad that describes the person you want. You don't want a nondescript ad that says, "Veterinary technician wanted." You'll get who knows what kind of person applying for an ad like that. You need to be really specific and start out by writing out what we call the 'ideal scene.' You need to write about this person that you're hiring like you already have them working in the clinic. Write down what they're doing, how they're helping you, how they're helping the practice. Where they fit in. Then you fashion an ad out of that.

Say for example, you need a veterinary assistant, someone that's going to help your technician. You want that person to be coachable. Your technician's going to be in charge of them and having them help her or him and they need someone that's not going to be giving them push back all day long and making their life more difficult when they're really supposed to be there to help them. You need someone who is willing and eager to learn. You need someone with a good attitude. You need someone that's decently smart. They've got to be *able* to learn. They have to be friendly.

All these things you should write out in your ideal scene-saying something like, "We have hired a veterinary assistant who everybody loves. She is very friendly, outgoing and she is positive. She comes in every morning on time with a smile on her face. She is willing to help wherever we need her. She is coachable. She listens to the instructions that we give and can follow them. She contributes to the practice by making clients feel comfortable, and greeting them in the hallways. She is keeping the rooms clean in between clients. She makes my staffs' jobs easier because of all of the things that she does. No job is too small or too big or too complicated. With proper training she can figure it out."

That would be your ideal scene and then based on that you're going to pick out the points that you want for your ad. For example, you could say, "Veterinary Assistant Wanted. (Practice name) is looking for an upbeat, positive team player who is willing to learn, follow directions and help out a hardworking team." That is just an example, you could add or subtract what you want based on that ideal scene. But that gives you an idea of what we're talking about. I think that is the important part, you need to know what you want and what you need before you even place that ad. If you don't, you're going to get candidates who apply that don't necessarily know what they want either. You have to be specific in your asking to get the right candidates to apply.

Once you have applicants for the position you need to do a few things. Number one is to review the resumes. Any red flag resume should be tossed out. They're really not worth spending your time interviewing. I'd consider a red flag if they've had 10 jobs in the last six years. They're not going to stay anywhere very long. Or if every job that they have listed on their resume since high school they've stayed at for three months, that tells you that either they're not a very good worker or, again, they're not happy wherever they are. You probably have your own list of red flags as well, and you can apply those at this stage of the game.

If they make that first cut then the next step that we take is what we call an aptitude test. Basically, it's a 'can you follow directions?' test. It's a simple two page test and it just gives us a grade that we can give the applicant, either passing or failing. This gives you an idea about their attention to detail and whether or not they will be able to follow instructions.

The next step following the aptitude test is a personality test. You could do an interview next, then the personality test. But I like to spend my time on candidates that I'm more inclined to hire so, if I spend 30 minutes interviewing them and then they fail the personality test they're not going to be someone that we would hire so I've just wasted that interview time. That's why I like to do the personality test first. There's a variety of different personality tests out there. Some of them are strictly online. You can buy some of those tests and then give the people login information to fill them out. You can work with consulting companies that have the tests and interpret them for you, and just call you with results. There's a variety of options, but you want to know a little bit about this applicant. For starters, you want to know they aren't some psychotic, truly crazy person. There may be really only two percent of the population that is truly antisocial and dangerous, but obviously that is something you would want to know, and those aren't the people you want working for you. There are other things that you can find out from this test also. If they are going to be covertly hostile they're not going to be good in a team environment. If they have issues going on in their life that are influencing them, you would want to know, because that will affect how they do their job. There really is quite a variety of things that you're going to find out and it definitely helps for selection of the right person for the job. You and your current staff should take the same personality test as well, so you know where you all fall on the spectrum. You will know what kind of person works for you and works best with you. This will help you just make a better selection, so that you're going to pick out someone that's going to fit well with the team versus clash at every turn.

After the personality testing and interpretation, as long as they're acceptable on that, move on to the interview. And the interview truly should be done by the team member this person will be working for. If you have someone on your staff that you want to duplicate, for example, if you have a great technician and you're looking for another technician, have that good tech start out interviewing the applicant. They're going to have a good feel for what they want and also how that person is going to help out at the clinic. We always say that if there's someone that you want to duplicate, have them do the hiring. That doesn't mean that you shouldn't review the personality test and probably take a few minutes to talk or interview them yourself but definitely have someone else talk to them, on the staff, that is doing a good job and is someone who you want more of. By all means, if you have a poor employee that you are trying to replaces, do not have them interview the new candidate.

There are a variety of techniques you can use during the interview. Usually just sitting down in a room with them, and talking, then asking a few pointed questions. I have a set list of questions that I go through, the same for each applicant, so you can compare answers. There will be a link at the end of the chapter containing our standard interview questions. This is just a good starting point. It gives you an idea where your applicant is at, and where they've come from. Of course they can lie to you. Hopefully on the personality test you found that out, if they aren't an honest person it's going to show up there. But, their answers will tell you a lot about their work ethic and preferences, and you can decide if they're going to work for you.

Depending on the position you are hiring for, your location, and the potential access to controlled drugs, you may also want to have a background check done on the applicants at this time. Depending on the personality test you use, ...

If you think they are looking good so far, don't commit either way yet. Sit down and talk to the staff that also interviewed them. Brainstorm on what you all liked or didn't like and how they would fit into the clinic. Then follow the interview up with scheduling a working interview. Pick a whole day or a half day where this person comes in and works alongside whoever it is for whatever position it is that you are hiring for. You may give them certain tasks based on the personality test also. For example, if their personality test said that they are great at starting projects but may have a hard time finishing them, you may want to give that person a list of tasks to do, show them how to do them, and then let them finish on their own. You'll be making sure that the follow through is something they can do. You don't want someone coming on board, starting everything and never finishing it. Or worst yet, telling you it's finished and you find out later that it's not. I recommend using a testing system where you can get a list of things like this to check for during the working interview.

If the working interview goes well, you can either schedule a second working interview or do a trial employment. With this, you tell the candidate that at the end of that period you will reassess to see if the job is working out on their end and see if they're performing the way you want them to. At that point you will come up with a plan for a permanent position or not, depending on both you and them. This gives both of you a way out if after 30 days you're thinking, "Gosh, this isn't going to work out." Or after 60 days, or anytime during that trial. You can pick a length of time that you feel works for you and your clinic. It can be whatever time period you're comfortable with. People can fake it for a certain amount of time, but they can't fake a good attitude and good performance for two months. So you're going to know what their true behavior is going to be like. You'll see how they're going work, and how they're going to work out with the rest of your staff. You'll see how they treat and interact with the clients. You'll know if the clients are going to like them, if that even matters in their position in the hospital. If they're a kennel person it probably doesn't have as big an impact on your decision. But, it's going to give you a good insight as to how they're going to perform over the long haul and their true personality.

That is our hiring protocol for finding new staff, now for existing employees. If you have team members that are working great this shouldn't be any type of awkward transition for them. They are likely already high performers: willing to work, excited about being there. They will fit right in with the new attitude of the clinic. However, if they aren't great performers or even if maybe you think they're doing fine but when you start implementing some of the ideas in this book all of a sudden they're pushing back saying, "No, I don't think I want to do that." "That's not a good idea." That will give you some more insight onto their true behavior and the way that they're going to fit with this new and improved clinic mentality.

In my experience, as you start to upgrade your clinic those people that aren't of the caliber that you need will naturally drop off. They're not going to want to hang with the people that are high performers, that are doing well, that are excited about showing their statistics (which we'll talk about in the next chapter). They're going to be the ones who fall off the wagon. They won't feel like they fit in anymore. They may be resistant to this change in little ways at first. As time goes on they might cause big scenes and put you through some drama before they finally admit that this isn't going to work for them. Or before you put your foot down and say, "You know what, it's not working out and we need to let you go."

But, your high performers are going to really enjoy the changes that you implement. They're going to want to play the games. They're going to want to be rewarded for their performance. They're going to want to show off how well they're doing too. That's the winning mentality that you really want and need in your clinic to keep everything moving forward. This kind of attitude will enable you to reach your goals, both for the clinic and personally.

PUT IT TO WORK

Now you have a general outline for getting new people into your employee pool using the right kind of ads, how to conduct the interview process, and some ideas about your current employees.

In the next chapter we'll talk about hats and stats and other things that will improve employee performance. When you implement these things is when you'll see how your current employees react to the changes. That's going to give you a good indicator about whether or not they're going to stay or go. And truly, if they're going to go, you are going to be better off without them. You'll be much farther ahead finding someone who has the attitudes of success that you want and need.

For a list of interview questions that will help you determine an applicant's appropriateness for your clinic, visit www.vetclinic-successsecrets.com/hire.

Chapter 3. Hats & Stats

"Problems are only opportunities in work clothes." - Henry J. Kaiser

Where Do I Belong?

So now you have your employees, what do you do with them? Everyone wants to know where they belong and how they fit in to the big picture. The same is true for your employees. By being clear on this, you are going to reduce confusion and give your staff ownership of their position. To have a team that works as a unit and smoothly flows from the front to back and vice versa, each person needs to know and own their position.

The Job

Each and every one of your employees has a certain job that you want them to do, and that job needs to have a written, all-inclusive description. This will tell them exactly what you expect of them and what they are supposed to do. And you give them this title and description when you hire them. This is called hatting. You are giving them the hat of "veterinary technician" or "lead receptionist." Your job descriptions need to be very detailed about what each person is responsible for and the things that they are in charge of. If they are under or over other people, this needs to be included as well, who they report to and who reports to them. All of this is essential to having your team own their 'hats.'

As far as the job description goes, this will let them know, without any confusion, what their number one priority is. This will tell them where they fit in, like a cog in a wheel, and that whole wheel is the smooth running veterinary clinic. Their cog is their portion of that, which is what they do to help everything run smoothly, the part that they're in charge of. If there's a problem in that area, it comes back to them. You can trace it back and address the issue. If something's going great, you can trace it back and find that it's them and give them the praise and the reward that they deserve for doing so well.

Each job, or each position in your practice needs to have a description and have a person who has been hatted with that description. You shouldn't hire someone and then find a position for them, you need to have a position and hire for that position. As a rule, that is what most of us do. For example, you may need two veterinary technicians, six veterinary assistants, and one or two receptionists. This is just an example, the case may be different in your clinic. You need to have a list of the positions that you have, and then make a specific description for each one. You may people that overlap positions, for example when your lead receptionist takes the day off, your assistant receptionist takes over that hat for the day. But each position need to have a title and a description, and a person to fill it.

If you already have team members in your practice, you need to be specific with them as far as the job description goes, and give them a hat. This may be a bit of a transition, but your goal is to have a position that anyone qualified can walk into and know exactly what they are supposed to do. This is creating systems to make your life easier in the future. Getting new hires up to speed won't be dependent on one person who 'has' to train all the new people coming in. This will make it easier on your existing staff when someone leaves, too. When you hire a replacement, it won't be entirely their responsibility to train the newbie. Of course they may have to help out and clarify any questions, but by and large it will be laid out for the new person in black and white.

As far as developing these descriptions on the fly, your staff can help you out with this. If you have someone in a position that is doing a good job, the way you want it done, give them a hat and then have them develop this job description. You may not know all that they do right now, but they do. They can go through what they normally do in a week and write those things down, so that you can then come up with the job description. You need to have all these descriptions in a clinic manual or handbook, where everything that happens in the clinic is documented. Not only everything that happens during the day, from the moment you walk in the door, but each job, each description, what each job is responsible for, and everything that goes on to make the clinic work like a well-oiled machine. And this leads me into our next topic, which is statistics.

Each position should also have a statistic, and that stat is measurable. The person whose job description is over that statistic will be responsible for that number. So for example, let's talk about your receptionist. She is responsible for booking the appointments. You could have her stat be the percentage of appointments booked. If you have 20 slots in a day and she had 18 filled, she's got a 90% for the day, and she can graph that. An essential part of having the statistic is actually keeping track of it and graphing it so you can track it over time. The idea is that you want those statistics to be going up. You don't want them to be flat. You don't want them to be going down. If they are headed in a downward trend, you can see that and you can address it before it's a bigger problem. You don't want to one day wake up and say, "Gosh, I have no appointments, what happened?" and then go looking. The whole idea behind the statistics that you're tracking is you're going to be able to spot trends before they get out of hand and you get to that day, when you wake up and there are no appointments.

An important part of the employee's job under their description is that they do have a statistic that's measurable. This makes it something that they can track themselves, and then present to you, so you know what is going on. You will know where they're at, how they're performing, and what's going on with each position. One important thing to remember about their statistic is that it has to be something they feel they have control over. If they don't feel like they have control, it's not going work. I've had other practice owners ask me, "How does the receptionist, have control over the number of appointments booked?" Well, believe you me, if she's answering the phone and that's her stat, she's going to be getting people in and filling up those appointment slots.

Not only is it unethical, and frankly illegal, to give medical advice over the phone, but it's not good practice, and it's not good medicine. Sometimes employees will try to 'help' people by giving them advice over the phone. This is something they should not be doing without consulting you. Because really you, as the veterinarian, are the only person that can give advice under a valid veterinary-patient-client relationship. This VCPR has to exist in order to dispense medicine or recommendations. I'm sure we've all had new clients call or people who are not even clients call to ask a question, and it may be tempting for the one answering the call to give advice. But this is not okay, and it's not good medicine. This is a perfect example of a time where the receptionist does have control. She can say, "We can't make any recommendations without seeing your pet, we need to have one of our doctors examine him. I can get you in at 10:30."

She is going to be motivated to get those appointments booked, not only those when people call for information, but even people that are price shopping. Anyone calling on the phone, including current clients, you can bet she's going to be more likely to get them in on the schedule if she's tracking that on a daily basis.

Keeping these stats, and having a stat for each position is vitally important because that makes sure that your staff is being productive in that position. If you have someone that doesn't want to keep track of their stats, or has a hard time graphing it, this can mean there's something going on there, something they aren't comfortable with. Either they don't want you to know because they're underperforming, or they don't feel like they have any control over their stat. It could also be they're giving you pushback because they don't like this new way of doing things. Make sure you show them how to track and graph it, so you know it is not a problem of mechanics. If the problem continues, you need to find the source of the problem and address it.

Keeping track of the statistics is very important for you to be able to monitor each position, and also to base bonuses and rewards on the basis of production. Because you want all the stats to be heading up, you need to reward each position for accomplishing that. If you have someone whose stat is going down, and everyone else's is heading up, or even normal, they're going to be dragging down the team, which means they're not pulling their own weight, and they truly don't deserve a bonus. You can't give blanket bonuses because then you're rewarding everyone, including those who aren't performing. If you do this, you are telling the whole team that it doesn't matter what your stats look like, good or bad, you'll get a piece of the pie. Then no one is going to take this seriously and take responsibility for their position. Or you'll have a great employee or two that keep trying and raising their stats in spite of the blanket bonus policy, but eventually they will get tired of this and leave your practice. And you will have lost the kind of employees you really need to keep. By basing bonuses on performance you are going to attract the kind of person that likes a challenge, knows you value them, and takes pride in their work. You don't want the under-performers taking anything away from those who are excelling at their job. This is a key aspect of hats and stats, rewarding performance based on stats.

It may take you a little while to figure out what a good statistic is for each position in your hospital, but it's worth taking the time and effort to go through the process and do it. Like I mentioned before, if you have someone who is super awesome at their position, talk to them, ask them, they're probably going to have a pretty good idea of what their stat should be. They can help you design how it should be measured for that position. And this will help you get on the road to making those stats for all the other positions as well. We used the example of the receptionist earlier, her stat being the number of appointments booked, and that is a great stat for a receptionist. If you have multiple receptionists, another stat might be the number of new clients booking appointments based on phone calls. Or the number of reactivated clients, who hadn't been in the clinic in the past year but now have an appointment booked due to a phone call or mailer.

Of course these are just examples, you may have a better idea of what you want your employees in each position to be doing and that what you want to be tracked. Part of designing all this is that you have your end goal in mind, you need to know what you want your practice to look like in the future. This will help shape these systems, so that as you're growing and making these positions and making the stats that go along with them, you're heading towards your goal.

All the doctors (including you!) need to have a stat also. Typically that's going to be production, how much you produced for the clinic during each working day. But it could be something else too. If you do a lot of the managerial work at the clinic and don't see as many appointments, maybe it's going to be how your ad is performing , or the number of new clients your marketing brought in. Or if you're filling all your positions that have been open, it could be hiring. Whatever you are comfortable with, and feel that you have control over. Remember, the same criteria apply to you! So it has to be something that's important to your position in the clinic, and something that's going to line up with your overall goals.

In conclusion, the hats that you're going to give your employees, and yourself, help everyone know exactly what their job is in the clinic. This tells them where they fit in, what their duties are, who they report to, and who reports to them. It is all going to be very clear and laid out, so there shouldn't be any confusion. And the nice thing is, if something comes up and there is confusion, you can address it, you can change the description, add or subtract something from that description. That way the next time you hire for that position, or the next time the policy is needed, there won't be any confusion about it. These are fluid things, and as your practice changes or grows into your master plan, you can adjust as needed. These may also change with the time of year, when there are different things going on as far as appointment schedule. For example, if you do beef cow work you know that in the springtime there's going to be a lot of calving calls. Or in February you are going to be scheduling a lot of dentals. So things are going to change a little bit based on that, and that's okay, you just have to plan for it, and know it's going to happen.

These statistics are important so that you can monitor everybody's contribution to the clinic and see how they're doing. You'll also get feedback from your employees. If they are all pushing, pushing, doing great, and there's somebody that's slacking and not doing their part, you're going to hear about that and you're going to see it reflected in that person's stats. We'll talk about this in Chapter 9, but when you go over these stats you'll do it in front of everyone, so everybody sees how the whole team is performing. This creates some peer pressure, which is good. It also allows you to see how everyone is performing and how that ties in with your week and your month and your year as far as how the clinic numbers look.

The Bottom Line

The whole idea of this chapter is having each of your employees knowing what their job is and how you are going to measure their performance it that job. This enables you to have performance-based rewards. Whether that's a monetary bonus, something big, or some special thing at the end of the year like a trip, or maybe even little weekly contests between the employees, you can track those things and reward them based on performance. That's how you're going to get and keep the top-performing employees- *by rewarding performance*. The high performers get rewarded, the ones that aren't performing won't like that, and they're going to drop out. Your clinic will be better off without them, and open those positions up so you can find motivated people.

The hats and stats are key to a smooth running clinic, and also to getting and keeping the kind of employees that you want and need to take your practice to the next level.

For an example of tracking and graphing the receptionist stats mentioned in this chapter, visit www.vetclinicsuccesssecrets.com/stats.

Chapter 4. Marketing Basics

"The aim of marketing is to know and understand the customer so well the product or service fits him and sells itself." - Peter Drucker

But Why?

Marketing. Funny, I don't remember taking a class on that in vet school... If you were smart, maybe you did in undergrad, but it's one of those things where the "if you build it, they will come," theory was implied. Kind of like that old baseball movie, which isn't always the case in our business. I don't know about you, but I have experienced that first-hand. We really should know at least the basics about marketing, because we *do* have to market ourselves.

I know some people think medical professionals shouldn't market themselves. It's unethical, or below us, or something like that. But, that truly is not the case. If you're going to compete in today's marketplace, you have to be able to market yourself. You have to be able to tell your potential clients why they should do business with you over all your competitors and over doing nothing. Because not taking their pet anywhere to receive medical attention is an option as well.

That's what this chapter on marketing basics is all about. So get rid of all your thoughts about, "I'm too good to do marketing," or, "I'm so good that I don't need to do marketing," or, "I have no idea what to do for marketing," because after reading this, you'll have a good idea about what you *should* do, at least as far as the basics are concerned. If you need help, there's always more help that can be found.

The Down & Dirty Basics

First off, don't worry. You don't have to pay some advertising person big bucks to make you a website and do your monthly advertising. I know when I've talked to companies that perform these services, they say, "$20,000" and they throw that number out there like, "Oh, I know you'll jump all over that," which isn't the case in my world. Maybe it is in yours, and if it is, more power to you, but do be careful, because some of those advertising agencies don't know the veterinary market. Or they don't know the true basics of marketing and what ads should do and what else is involved besides ads in marketing *your* practice to *your* ideal customer.

Let's start first with your physical building, assuming most of you have a sign out front. Don't be fooled that your sign has to be beautiful and pretty and catchy. All it has to do is let people know where you are. If they're driving and they're coming to see you, they're already looking for you. You want them to be able to find you. You want them to be able to read the letters and the words that are on the sign. You have probably driven to s business before, and knew you were going to a business at a certain address, and yet were unable to find it on the first or maybe even the second or third pass. The sign may be written in a font that is illegible, the colors may be wrong, or you can't see it from the road. So keep all that in mind when you are designing and putting up your sign. Or if you already have a sign, get some fresh eyes and look at it to see if it's doing its job.

If it's not, don't freak out about it. If you're on a major road or a street that people frequent, you do need to have a sign, because some people will come and visit you, just based on seeing your business at that location. Your sign should also have your phone number on it if so those people see your sign and want to call, they can. Beyond a clearly visible sign with your name that tells the reader what kind of business you are in and your phone number, you can do what ever you would like. Just be sure you aren't hiding the business and phone number behind a bunch of words that are so busy they become distracting.

Secondly, in this day and age, you do have to have an Internet presence. I'm sure you're all aware of that. You should have a website. You should have a Facebook account, and depending on your clientele and where you're located, there may be a need for some of the other social media options. The minimum online presence you should have would be Facebook and a website. I also am a firm believer in still maintaining an ad in the physical yellow pages. Unless you're in an area where there are very few older people (baby boomers and older) you're going to want that because those people still use the phone book. And those baby boomers control most of the discretionary income in our society. Some younger people may not even know what the yellow pages are, but the older people definitely use the phone book. And you might be pleasantly surprised at how much business you'll get from a good ad in the yellow pages.

Another key thing about this marketing is you need to track where people are coming from. So when you have new clients come in, one of the questions that you need to ask them has to be, "How did you hear about us?" You need to track those responses. If it's the Internet, was it your website or Facebook or a different site? If it's the yellow pages, you want to know that. If it's physical location, if it's from a friend or a referral from a client, these are all things that you need to know.

Tracking is one of the strict rules of marketing. You have to know your return on investment for each type of ad. Before you renew your yellow pages ad each year, you need to get a quote from the yellow pages salesperson, and then look up on your computer system by source how many new clients and the amount they spent that was generated from that ad in the past year. That will tell you what the ROI is on that particular media. It's simple math. You take what you invested divided by the return and you want each type of advertising you do to at least bring in as much as you spent. What you would really like to see is 1:2 or even higher. Another thing that you can incorporate into that math is the lifetime value of a client. You may have an expensive advertising media, but it brings you really great clients. Track those clients, and if their lifetime value is high enough, it may justify less than a 1:1 ROI the first year. This lifetime value of a client is a number that you should know. You can track an average for your entire clientele, and then get more specific with certain sources of clients. With computer software this is a pretty easy number to figure to find and track.

So the three basic places you should have a presence are your physical sign, the paper yellow pages, and the Internet, via your website and Facebook. Depending on what kind of work you do, there may be other places that your name can be found as well. For example, if you have a CO_2 laser, a lot of times the Surgical Laser Society will list your clinic on their website. So if people are specifically looking for laser surgery, your name shows up. And there's going to be different locations, virtual and physical, depending on what you do, the equipment you have, and the area you live in. Talk to the manufacturers or the distributors of the equipment you use, and see if there is somewhere else that your name and your clinic can be listed. Anywhere, and everywhere, really, that your clinic name is out there is good, because somebody will see it. Someone will be looking for something, and you'll show up.

For targeted advertising, you need to figure out who your ideal client is. For this, a great exercise is to sit down with pen and paper, either just you, or you and one of your receptionists, or you and your whole team, and talk to them and brainstorm about who your ideal clients are. You probably have one or two current clients that came to mind as soon as you heard the words, "ideal client." You may have thought, "Oh gosh, that's Mrs. Jones." Well, let's talk about Mrs. Jones… How old is she? What kind of animals does she have? How many does she have? What does she do? What are her hobbies? Where are her friends? All these answers are going to give you good ideas about where you need to be in your marketing to show up where those people are. Continue this exercise by writing a biography about your fictional ideal client. This is a good paragraph to review before you place any new ads, write any mail pieces or plan any new marketing campaigns.

What your goal needs to be with your marketing is to show up everywhere your ideal client is. If you live in a community where there's a golf course, and your ideal clients typically are golfers, then figure out how you can get your name there. Can you sponsor a hole? Can you do provide something in the goody bag for a tournament? Can you have an ad in the clubhouse? You could really dive in depth on this after you have your ideal client pinned down.

Another useful piece of marketing is direct mail. You have a few options here, one is 'every door direct mail' through the US Postal Service. If there are certain neighborhoods that your clients live in, you can target just those neighborhoods. You can target that zip code or a certain mail route. This is easy to look up on the United States Postal Service website. It will show you the routes in your area (or any area), tell you how many people are on each route, how many of those are residences, how many are businesses and what the median income is. It'll give you a lot of information, and it's a cheap and easy way to reach those people.

There are different campaigns that you can mail to them. You could do just a simple postcard. You could do a series of letters, and some of it depends on who they are. If it's a high-end neighborhood, you're going to want to do a high-end mailing. So that might be a fancy envelope with a nice letter written on thick paper, not just the plain white paper you pull out of your printer. These are things you can have printed off either at your local copy store, or you can order them online. You have a lot of options for this. Later we'll get a little more into the details of what your mail pieces need to have in them to get a response.

Obviously you don't want to ignore your current clients in search of new ones, so you need to have part of your marketing plan be how you're going to keep in contact with them. In this plan you'll need to have offers for them and things you do for them to keep you at the top of their mind. That way, there's no doubt that when they have a problem, you are the only one they're going to call. Or when their friend has an animal problem, they're going to say, "You have *got* to call *my* vet." We'll talk about this more in the promotions chapter too, but staying at the top of their mind for your clients is essential. It's not their job to remember that you're there. It's your job to remind them that you're there, so that when something comes up, they're going to call you.

Part of your marketing plan also needs to be a referral program. When we were talking about tracking where your clients come from, one of those tracking options needs to be a client referral. And you need to know who the client is that referred them, because you're going to want to thank them. Some of you already do this, and that's great. That's awesome! People love it, and I would challenge you to not only thank them by sending them a card, giving them a credit, sending a gift card, or something along those lines - whatever you want. But to also put their names on a list or spreadsheet, and when they start referring more people, when they have a second referral, they get treated differently. They get more special stuff. They get something great and they think, "Gosh, I wonder what they're going do next?" So they refer someone else. What happens the third time they refer someone? You could even do a drawing for people that refer a certain number of clients, new clients, in a specific time period. You need to find out what a new client is worth to you, monetarily. Figure out your average transaction for new clients, and the average annual value of those clients. You might be surprised by that number. Then, based on this number, come up with a really cool gift that you can offer as a drawing prize. Make it a game.

Say you have a contest for each quarter, and if you refer three new people, then your name is entered in a drawing. That drawing could be for an iPad or a weekend getaway or something else kind of big. You'll be surprised what the referred new client is worth, especially over the course of a year, let alone the lifetime of a pet. By knowing this number, it will give you the power to say, "I can reward these people by doing the iPad, doing the weekend getaway," whatever it is you think that your clients would enjoy. Maybe a round of golf at that nice golf club, whatever! Something that's going to be a high perceived value to them and will keep them referring their friends. Only now, they've got even more reason to make those referrals.

Then make a big deal out of the winner. Make it huge, lots of attention. Do the drawing on Facebook live and publish it in your newsletter. Get those people the recognition they deserve.

One more thing that you should focus energy on is reviews. Encourage people to leave reviews on Google and on Facebook, even on your website. You can put a little form in there that they can fill out to leave a review. You want to know what they're thinking, and you need this for a couple of reasons:

If it's something great, which I hope the vast majority are, you want other people to read that. We live in a day and age where social proof is huge. So if you have a whole bunch of five-star reviews and the other clinics in town have one or two or none because they're not putting much effort into it, then you're going to be way ahead. On the flip side, if it's not something good, you want to be able to address that. You want to have a chance to rectify it. And most of all, you want to know about it. Maybe there is something in the flow of your office you can improve, or maybe there is one particular incident or employee that was the source of the problem. Sometimes, it's nothing you or your staff did, but that person was not going to be happy no matter what. Just like in life, that is going to happen. Nowadays, most people are on the Internet, and people love to comment about their visit and leave reviews. It somewhat depends on where you live. There are some small towns where that's is not a high priority for the clientele, and they would much rather rely on word of mouth. If you live in a place like that, you need to know it and have a plan to get people talking about you. We will address that in the next chapter, too.

TAKE ACTION

These truly are just the basics. Basic things that you should have going on in your clinic so that you have your name out there. These things will keep a steady stream of new clients walking in the door. Existing clients also have the option to refer and be acknowledged and cheered for doing that. These ideas will also help you know where to advertise and what the purposes of your ads are.

If you have competing clinics nearby, this gives you the upper hand. Everything you can do along these lines, all these different ways you can show up to your clients and potential clients, is going to make you stand out and be the place where people go.

To get more a checklist of what every ad must have, go to
www.vetclinicsuccesssecrets.com/ads

Chapter 5. Keep in Touch

"Eighty percent of success is showing up." - Woody Allen

Be Memorable

Have you ever hired a serviceman, had a good experience, and never heard from them again? Chances are, the answer is yes. Think back on one of these instances, and try to come up with the name of the person or company. Can you remember? I had this experience just the other day. Our architect who is helping my husband and I design our remodel needed the survey with elevations to put with the house plans. For the life of me, I couldn't come up with the name of the company who did the survey. The sad thing is, we had hired the same company several years before to do the survey before construction began on our clinic. I had multiple positive experiences with this company, but the only time I heard from them was when *I* called them. And with my memory the way it is, I may just call up some other company by mistake. What a lost opportunity on their part to follow up with someone who had used their services, had a good experience, and based on past history, is likely to need their services again. If you don't want to be like this company, who may lose a good, paying customer, not because I was unhappy, just because I forgot about them, you need to take a look at your clinic's system for keeping in touch with clients. Sometimes we take ourselves as veterinarians too seriously. We think that because we did what was expected, we deserve all future business from our clients. This thinking will only get you so far, and with a small percentage of people. It is your responsibility to 'wow' your client with a good experience, and then to keep reminding them that you are still here and waiting to provide more services when they are ready. Don't let those clients go somewhere else next year, just because they never heard from you and then forgot about you.

THE POWER OF SHOWING UP

Keeping in touch with clients is very important. Like I have mentioned previously, you need to stay at the top of their mind. It's not their job to remember you. It's your job to remind them that you're there so that you are the one they call whenever something is needed. There are a variety of ways to do this, to keep in touch with them, and probably the most effective ways are print newsletters, emails and Facebook posts. If you do a monthly newsletter, a weekly email, and frequent Facebook posts, you will really keep your clinic at the top of your client's mind and remind them that you're there for them whenever they need you. I know you've probably all heard that you *should* do monthly newsletters or do a clinic newsletter, and some of you do, and that's awesome. If you don't do this, you can't realize the power of it until you start, and the connection that people develop with you because of it.

In those newsletters you can talk about a variety of topics. Make some of it fun, though. Don't make it all educational. People do want to learn, but more than that, they want to be entertained. You can put recipes in your newsletter. You can put in funny stories or cartoons. You can have a monthly column that someone from the clinic writes. It could be something off-the-wall or funny, or some kind of a 'Dear Abby' column, or whatever you can come up with. Survey your clinic team to see what you've got talent-wise, and be sure that somebody can commit to doing it every month.

Another way to make the newsletter personal is to highlight different employees and doctors every month. That way your clients are getting to know your staff versus their brief conversation when they come in for an appointment. There's probably not a lot of personal conversation going on, which is good, because you want your employees to be efficient when they're working. And your technicians in the back may not have any or very little contact with the clients. But your clients do want to know about you and your staff personally. It's human nature. They also want to know who is caring for their pet. People are curious about people, and so when you're doing these profiles for your staff members or for yourself, make it fun.

Make it a brief synopsis of where they came from, what their current life is like, what they like to do, and then also put some fun stuff in there. Something like 'three things Dr. Jeff wishes he had never done,' or 'three things you might not know about Annie.' Items of interest like that where people will be intrigued and it's something they can talk about or mention the next time they come in. "Gosh, I never knew you used to ride big wheels," or whatever the subject was. That makes them feel like they know you, and people do business with people that they know, like, and trust. So that's something that builds affinity and friendliness. It builds that camaraderie where they feel like they know you.

In your newsletter, you can also talk about any promotions you have going on. We will talk more about promotions in the next chapter. You can feature your upcoming event, or in-office special. Or there may be some other community event that is somehow related to animals or veterinary medicine or to your clinic or to people inside your clinic. Those are human interest stories, and people really enjoy these. You can also look up fun dates, official holidays this month or fun dates to remember for the month. You can look up what national holidays there are like, 'bring your cat to work day' or 'national walk your dog day.' Things like that people will get a good laugh out of or a 'Gee Whiz' when they read.

You also have an opportunity with this newsletter to make it a part of your referral program. So you're encouraging clients to refer people (and you're tracking those referrals!) not only so you know where they came from but also track how much money they brought in. I think you'll be pleasantly surprised each month to see how much business client referrals bring in. Those tend to be your best clients because they're like your current clients, and as a rule those are the people that embody your ideal customer. In your newsletter, you can mention all of the clients that referred people last month, new clients. Everybody loves to see their name in print. You're sending this newsletter out to all your clients, and the clients who referred people to you last month (who are special people who help bring more business/money to your practice) are getting recognition. They love that. It makes them feel good. It's good for you to mention it. Other people may see their friends' names in there and think, "Gosh, I'm going to refer someone so I get my name in the newsletter, too."

You could even highlight something. If you have dental month coming up, do an interview with an owner whose dog hadn't been feeling well because of dental disease. You performed this successful dental, pulled teeth, worked your magic, and now that dog is doing great. We all have stories like this in our clinic. Call those owners up and ask if you can interview them for your next newsletter. Stories like those hit home with people because they can relate. This is another client who's just like them, they didn't know what was going on with their pet. They brought it in and the problem was fixed, and, wow, now the dog is doing great. That's a good way to point out things that they might not think about with their pets mouth, if it's dental month, or relating to any other special you have coming up, promotion-wise. Find some problem or disease that relates to what you want to focus on and talk to people. People, like I said, want to have their name in print. They enjoy that. They want to help other pet owners, too, and some of them may say, "Wow, I had no idea bad teeth could make my dog so sick." Chances are if they think that, a lot of other people, a lot of your other clients think this, too. It's a good opportunity for you to educate in way that uses social proof and tells a story. You're talking to another client who was just like the client reading the newsletter, and they learn these things and now their pet is doing great, and that's really what all your clients want. A nice, healthy pet. They want you to help them get there. They may not know how to get there, but that's why they come to you, and this newsletter is an opportunity for you to educate them indirectly.

The beauty of an interview or a story is that you're not sitting down and telling them about it individually. Although you can do this, and should do this in the exam room (which is another great opportunity location), but you're going to reach a lot more people with this newsletter. Maybe you didn't see the person reading the newsletter in the past few months, or maybe they only came in to buy food or flea prevention and didn't have a chance to talk to one of the doctors. Now they're going to have a chance to read this when it shows up in their mailbox (because you're showing up in their world!), and they're going to pay attention to it.

As you can see, there are a lot of opportunities and different ways to use this newsletter. It can be as short or as long as you want it to be. It could be as simple as one page front and back that has all the different things you want to talk about in there. It could be four pages where it's 11" by 17" and folded, and you can fill these with pictures, longer articles, and in-depth stories. It is usually pretty easy to find a local printer, maybe even one of your clients, who can print this out each month. You can get a spreadsheet of names and addresses of your current clients from your practice software. Then either print labels and stamp these yourself, if your staff has the time, or find a mailing house that has this process automated.

So, that's the newsletter. The next step is emails, and weekly emails are a good frequency. So this is only four to five emails per month, which isn't too much for someone to receive and isn't too much for someone to write either. These emails should have some sort of a call to action. So have a promotion or a special going on that month, give your clients a reason to come into the office. That's what these emails need to focus on. Maybe the call to action is referring a friend. Maybe it's coming in to get their free, engraved, personalized tag when they bring their pet in for vaccines. Whatever the special is, make this email something that's going to get them motivated to take action. Educational emails are fine, and I think they do have a place, but you need to have a once a week email that asks them to do something. You want that client to take action, and this email's job is to convince them to do it.

I'll provide some examples for you at the end of the chapter that you can look at, but it really doesn't take all that much time. If you sit down perhaps at the end of the previous month, commit an hour to two hours to this, get them all done, and get them scheduled. So part of this is also your client management software. You need to collect emails on clients, and then you need to have some kind of a system to keep in contact with them. You may have veterinary software that can email. I know some systems send out emails for appointment reminders. See if yours has the capability to send out broadcast emails. If not, there are plenty of other computer programs or applications that are available to do this. There's Constant Contact, Infusionsoft, and many others. AWeber is the one that our clinic uses. It's pretty simple to use, and you can import a spreadsheet of your client names and emails. There is also ClickFunnels, and many other different computerized options for doing this. Don't get overwhelmed with the technical part. Chances are, someone on your staff can do it if you don't feel comfortable. This can be an important part of your marketing and a great tool to use to keep in touch with your clients.

There will be a certain percentage of your clients that don't use email, and that's okay. They may not even have an email address, and that's all right, too. There will be another percentage that reads their emails religiously every day, and anything you send them they're going to respond to. Those are your tech-responsive clients. They are going to love having you keep in contact with them via their preferred method of communication.

There are also several other options you can choose from as far as keeping in frequent contact with your clientele. My third basic recommendation would be Facebook posts. Just have the posts frequently enough that people see you and see your clinic, and know what you do. There will be a percentage of your clients, again, who are not going to be on Facebook, and that's okay. You don't need them to be there. You'll reach them with one of the other modalities of contact that you're using. But the ones that use Facebook are very interactive with it. They're going to comment on your posts. They're going to like all your posts. They're going to ask questions.

Whatever you can do to get your clients engaged in whichever media they prefer is great, because again, you're staying at the top of their mind and showing up in their world. When their friend bemoans, "My dog is not feeling well," they're going to say, "Oh, you have to go see my vet," because earlier that same day they were on your Facebook page or reading your email or print newsletter. They remember your name.

THE WHY AND HOW

There's big advantages to staying in front of your clients all the time, not only for increasing visits, but for the referrals it's going to generate. Once again, be sure you track the business brought in each month by category. On your new client form, be sure to ask them how they heard about you. Look at these each month after implementing these strategies to see the difference it makes in your bottom line. Also pay attention to your monthly specials or promotions, and see how they increase as well.

Check out some sample emails at www.vetclinicsuccesssecrets.com/email.

Chapter 6. Promotions

"I believe that if life gives you lemons, you should make lemonade... And try to find somebody whose life has given them vodka, and have a party." - Ron White

The Happy Client

We all know there is nothing like a happy client telling everyone they know about your clinic. Just imagine seeing a client the day after a fun event, and they are thanking you for inviting them to the party and telling you how much fun they had. Are they going to be coming back in time and time again? You know it! And they are going to tell all their friends how great your place is. What better way to build loyalty and garner attention than to have fun events for your clients and their friends to attend? It's easier than you think to plan and execute fun promotions that make your clients love you and are great team builders for your employees.

What to Plan?

One idea for a fun promotion or event at your clinic would be to have a book signing. See if there are any local authors that have new books out, or maybe you have a client that has authored a book. Find a book that is animal related or agriculture related, something you think your clients might be interested in... maybe wildlife, local history, pet stories or something along those lines. You can host the author at your clinic, have them bring in books that people can buy and then have signed. You could also provide some snacks for the party. Try to find a client that does catering, or if there's a local shop, café, or bakery that does some small catering have them do the job. You will be involving other businesses or clients, which is always a good idea, and it will be a fun, social opportunity for your clients. Do what you can to get people involved so that they want to come out. They will have fun! It becomes a social event, and it's not just that they call when their animals are sick or when they need vaccines, but they think of you as a part of the community. They're seeing you in a different light. They're also seeing friends and other acquaintances that they may have and maybe people they know but didn't know were clients of yours also, and there's another connection. Another link to you, that will keep you at the top of their mind and keep them coming back.

Everything that you can do to build loyalty and make a deeper bond between you and your clients is practice building. If you stay in front of them all year long, then when there's a problem they're going to come back to you. There's no question in their mind. They're not going to go through the phone book or see who's cheapest or closer. They're going to know you, both personally and professionally, like you, trust you, and you're going to be the veterinarian that they come to when they have a problem. You're also going to be the vet they recommend and talk about to their friends and acquaintances.

Another fun idea, and one that we utilize in our clinic every year, is an Open House. The whole clinic is cleaned and spotless, top to bottom. It takes several weeks to get ready. Everybody, in their spare time, is cleaning everything, making it beautiful. If you're going to show the clinic off, you want it to look amazing. Plan some fun things for people to do while they are there. Let them come during the day and walk through the clinic. You need to have set hours for the event, which tends to group people closer together, versus them trickling through all day long. Make some baskets to raffle off and have giveaway items as well, some fun things that people can just pick up and take with them. Call your sales reps and distributors and see what they have for freebies. For the baskets, you can sell raffle tickets with the proceeds benefitting a local animal cause. Most of your clients are going to like to support animal charities, so they feel good buying these raffle tickets. You can make different themed gift baskets that they can enter their raffle tickets in to win. This is also a great place to get your staff involved. You'll find some of them are social planners and love this kind of thing. And that will make your part even easier! This is also something you can promote on Facebook, your clinic website, your monthly newsletter, and the local paper. You could even have the drawings on Facebook live for your raffle. There are a lot of options here with social media as well as traditional media to get your clinic some attention and local press. Call a local reporter and let them know what you are doing. They might just show up!

Here are some ideas for fun things to do at an open house: you can have a barbecue. Put up a sign, "For a $5 donation, get a burger or hotdog, chips and a soda…" once again, the proceeds going to your charity of choice. You could have a dog wash. Supply the shampoo and hose(if it is summer!) in a plastic kiddie pool, and let the owners and your staff give Fido a bath. Have some sort of competition or event the dogs can try out- like a frisbee toss or agility course. You can have a variety of things going on at the same time that your staff and your friends help out with, and put your family to work as well. Promote all of this as "Come and meet us, walk through the clinic. See all the things that we have, the services we offer, and support this great charity at the same time." People really go for that.

You could even do two phases of the open house- the general one open to the public, and a VIP one for your best clients. Combine them on the calendar, so you can prepare for both of them at the same time. Have the VIP version the night before or the night after the daytime, open-to-the-public one.

Make the VIP one special, make it for your really good clients. The names on that list may or may not be the same every year, but start by looking at your top 100 clients. Who spent the most money this year? Go through that list. See who you want to invite. Plan something fun. You could either have the event at your clinic and let them walk through and have a chance to enter the raffles, or you could rent a space someplace nearby if your clinic doesn't lend itself to this kind of thing.

There's a lot of good ideas for this one, the options are endless! You could have a local band come out and play. You could have a local winery come out to do tastings. You can have basically anything you can think of, but make it something special for those good clients so they can come and see you on a social level. Again, that's something that builds the bond between them and you and your clinic, and it's kind of a reward for them, too. A lot of people really like that. They want to be treated special. They love their animals. They're spending a lot of money on them. They like to be recognized for that. Right here are a couple events that people are going to love. It's going to be something that they really enjoy, and that most your competition does not do. One more thing to set you apart.

One last promotional idea for an event to get your clients involved with your clinic is a pet food drive. Some of you may already be doing this, and I applaud you. Christmas or Thanksgiving would be a perfect time for this. It's the season of giving. People are in the mood for that, and you could have a pet food drive for one of your local shelters or animal rescue groups. Again, you must pick one that does a good job. You know who they are. You know which ones don't do a good job. Pick one that *does* a good job. Promote it to your clients. Maybe they get something special. They get a gift if they bring in a donation, or they get 5% or 10% off their bill. Whatever it is, make it something fun, and then also really push that promotion so that you're getting your clients involved. Set a goal. Say "We want to collect 1,000 pounds of cat and dog food for our shelter! Please help us do that." When you call people to remind them of their appointments, tell them again that you're having this pet food drive. Encourage them to bring something in, and give them some type of reward for doing it. Then, at the end, tally everything up. Make a big deal about it, how much food we gathered, and it's going to this shelter or cause. Maybe call a local paper, a local reporter. See if they want to come over when you give all of it to the shelter. When you present it, you can drive it over in the back of a van or a truck (make a big deal out of it), or you could have the shelter come to your clinic to pick it up. While the reporter is there, get some pictures. This is something to promote what you do, something that tells the community your clinic is involved, and you care, and you're supporting local causes with their help. They're like a team member when you're doing this. They're on board. They helped raise this gift, and they're going to be excited. They're going to enjoy seeing the fruits of their labors, the smile on the shelter director's face when they see all that you collected for them. They want to be a part of something bigger and to know that it's going to a good cause.

The bottom line is that your clients want to know that you care, and you're involved. That is something important for us to remember. I'm sure you've heard the quote "They don't care how much you know, until they know how much you care." It's not just that we do a good job, but that the community perception is that we are involved, that we've got a stake in this community. Which, of course, we do, because the people that live here are providing our living and our employees' living. I think sometimes, we think that people just know about our involvement, or understand it or expect it, but that's not always the case. Especially in cities where you can be anonymous. We *do* have to promote ourselves. And there is nothing wrong with that! We have to let people know what we're doing that's good. If you help out a shelter with surgeries, or if you donate certain procedures, or you treat shelter animals, make that known. People really like that. They want to know that you're involved, that you care, and that those things that are important to them are important to you, also.

For most pet owners, shelters or animal rescues are big touchpoints. Our clients, for the most part, have soft hearts. That's why they have these animals they are bringing to us in the first place. That's why they're bringing them to you to take care of, because they want the best for them. And they have a really soft spot for those animals that don't have homes. They want to do what they can to support those causes. Whatever you can do, event-wise or promotion-wise, that involves the less fortunate animals is going to get attention from your clients. It's going to get attention from the media, too. You can even call one of your local news stations and see if you can get on their show and talk about your event and who it is benefitting. Especially around Christmas time, they're always looking for feel-good stories, and it's easier than you think to get on local TV. If you call up the morning show host and tell them what you're doing and ask if you could come tell their audience about it, most of them are going to say 'yes.' If you're having a hard time getting on, tell them you'll bring a puppy or a kitten! It seems like that's always a good ticket to get yourself seen, something cute and fuzzy that you can bring with you when you go. Borrow a kitten or puppy from the shelter your event is supporting.

If you get in with one of these TV reporters, or you know one of the morning show hosts or the lunchtime host, they're going to be willing to have you come back for other things, too. If you have other events going on, like your open house or the book signing or anything like that, they'll be willing to have come back to their show. You can also offer your services as an expert so that if there is something going on in the community, like an animal event, a county fair, or on the darker side, if some kid develops an E. Coli infection after visiting a petting zoo. In situations like that you can utilize your connection with that TV host and be the expert guest.

The more you're seen, the more rapport you're going to build with people. Not only your clients, but people that see you on TV and then say "Wow, I'm going to go to that veterinarian's clinic. They must really know what they're talking about." They'll say this because you're on TV, you're the guest expert. They'll like what you are promoting.

This is just another great way to stay in front of your audience, in front of your pet owners, not only the ones that are currently your clients, but the ones that are potential clients and may bring their animals in just because they see you…everywhere!

TOP OF MIND

These are just a few ideas that you can use to stay in front of your clients. These things will get your clients involved, and help you to stay in touch with them throughout the year so that they don't only think of you once a year when their pet needs vaccines and they get a postcard. You can use these events to educate people as well, about the value of annual and semi-annual checkups, local concerns, etc. And there are so many more ideas out there! Ask your staff, they may have some great input and new ideas that would work really well in your community and with your clientele. They also want to be valued, and asking their opinion and getting them involved is a great way to show how much you appreciate them!

The bottom line is that part of your job is to remind your clients about who you are, what you stand for and that you are the one they need to come to for their animals. Don't expect them to remember, or always think of you, make it your goal to have your name be the automatic response to any animal concern.

For some great ideas of items to raffle at your Open House, visit www.vetclinicsuccesssecrets.com/raffles. **Lots of examples are included in the guide.**

Chapter 7. All About Clients

"The best way to look at any business is from the standpoint of the clients." - Jamie Dimon

Your Lifeblood

In this chapter, we're going to talk about clients. That is who pays your paycheck, your staff's wages, pays for your kids education and your vacations. They are the lifeblood of your clinic. Without them, you don't have a business. So treating them right and keeping them (new and old) coming through the door has got to be your primary focus. So we're going to address how to get new clients, offer more ideas about how to keep your current clients as raving fans, and how to maximize the lifetime value of your clients. Most of us want to grow our businesses and what we most commonly think about along those lines is acquiring new clients. Don't get me wrong, new clients *are* important for growing a business, but don't overlook the importance of your current clients during advertising campaigns. We're not going to focus all our energy on just acquiring new clients, because if we can keep more of your old ones coming in, your growth will be more steady and predictable. All three of these aspects of the client lifecycle are essential and will be addressed in this chapter.

The Good Stuff

We will start off with several ways to attract new clients to your clinic. The first and most important is your referral program. We've talked about that several times so far. You want to do everything you can to encourage your current clients to refer new clients to you. This includes handing out cards when new clients are at the office for any appointments or services, and welcome letters to new clients. These letters let them know that if they're happy with your services, you would love for them to refer their friends. It should also tell them about how you offer a rewards systems for referrals.

First of all, the cards that you can hand out to clients at their visits should look like and be about the size of a business card. We call ours 'care to share' cards and you can call yours whatever you like, but it's something that all the staff knows is a referral card. You give these out to your clients, and it's something easy that they can carry with them in their wallet or their purse. The next time they're talking to a friend or an acquaintance, and somebody says they need to find a vet, or their animal has some sort of special need, your client can say, "Oh, my vet gave me this card," and hand your card to that person.

They've got it in their purse, it's small enough to fit there, they hand it over and it gets the person they give it to a free exam. A free *first* exam, so it can't be a current client, but is made for new clients. The person that handed it out also gets a ten dollar credit to their account. It's a rewards system for both the new client and the current client who has referred someone.

You need to track these referrals so that you know if there are certain people that keep referring. If a client gives you a second referral, you need to do something special for that client. They have shown themselves to be a frequent source of referrals, and that's a really valuable client. That's someone you want on your side. For example, you could send them a letter saying how great it is to have clients like you. Thank you for your referral, and send it with a small box of chocolates from a local chocolatier, or someplace that makes goodies people really like and enjoy. This client gets a special reward for making multiple referrals. If they refer a third time, then you need to have an escalating program that you implement for these people. That way you know who's referring, you reward them appropriately and it will come to a point where they keep referring people, not only because they love you, but also to see what you're going to do next to surprise them. It's a fun game and clients enjoy that.

When you do have new clients come in, always send out a welcome card. Put a picture of their animal on it and the whole office team signs it and that goes out within the first week after seeing the new pet. We do this for new clients, and we also do it for existing clients when they get a new pet. So we have either a welcome card or a congratulations card. Congratulations on your new addition or welcome to our family are the two separate cards. Then after a couple weeks, send out a letter and this letter talks about their first visit, "We hope you had a great visit. We'd love to hear feedback from you. If you had a great experience, we want you to share that with your friends. Here are a couple cards" and include a couple of those 'care to share' cards in that letter and it's signed by the owners of the practice and it goes out in the mail to those new clients.

Those new clients are also put on our newsletter mailing list, so sometime within the first month after they've come in for their first visit, they will receive our printed newsletter. We ask for email addresses on our new client form, so we can put them into our email system as well, and they start getting the weekly emails that the clinic is sending out. There's also a welcome and informative series of emails that they'll be registered for as well. Those come out on a different schedule, it's not a weekly basis like our promotional emails are.

You should have a first in the series email that's a welcome email and it tells them how glad you are to have them coming to your practice and be a part of your practice family. It also tells them how to connect with you on Facebook, gives them your web address, and their options for emergency services. Give them your phone number, tell them if there is a different after hours phone number, and give them any special instructions or special information that you want all your clients to have. This can and should also be given out in a new client package that they receive at the time of their first visit. Now you're reaching people both ways, both in print, something they take home from their visit and as an electronic follow up reminder that they can always look up in their email if they lose the paper. Or, like I mentioned previously, some people are technology people, some people are not and either way, you're going to reach them. They can hold it in their hand and read it, or they can look it up on the computer and read it, but they're going to get that information from you.

I think it's a great idea to have a welcome package that you give your new clients and you can either do that at the time of their first visit or a couple days later, you could send them something in the mail. It would be a small package versus just a letter, and that's even better. Everyone loves receiving something unexpected, and that's something that people are going to remember. It's going to stand out. You could even include your welcome card in that package and maybe include some branded material from your clinic. It could be a coffee mug, or a leash with your clinic name on it, or a collapsible water bowl for dogs, a cat toy for cats. The bottom line is make it something that's fun for them and fun for their pet, something that's going to really make you stand out and bond with them.

This doesn't take a whole lot of effort on your part. You'll print out the personalized picture and card, obviously, but everything else can be standard for a dog or for a cat or for an exotic, depending on what type of animals you see. You can tailor this package to your business, and by including your branded items it becomes a personal gift. It's your business that has this special thing that you're sending out to your clients.

Now, where are these new clients going to come from? That's where your marketing comes in handy and your advertising. There are different ways you can accomplish this. There's a direct mail service provided by the USPS called Every Door Direct Mail, which we talked about in chapter 4. There's advertisements in the paper. Sponsorship of local events. All the places that you show up are going to be places that new people can see you.

Let's move on to existing clients. As mentioned before, if one of your current clients gets a new animal, always send them a congratulations card, something acknowledging the new addition to the family, something that lets them know that they're appreciated. A lot of what you can do for your existing clients, we have gone over already. Part of that is keeping in touch with them about your special promotions, your open house, your client appreciation events, or fun thing that you sponsor and put on for your clients.

You also want your clients to know everything that you offer service wise, so that they don't think mistakenly think they need to go find these services elsewhere. You don't want them to one day (after they've been a client for five years) say, "Wow, I didn't know you have a groomer!" You want to be clear and up front with them, letting them know all that you do. Once again, this is your responsibility to tell them, not theirs to just know. If you have a groomer on staff or that comes and works out of your clinic, you want to advertise that. You want your clients to know that. If you have special reproductive services, you want to make sure that all your clients with intact animals or your clients who are breeders are aware of that. You want them to know if there're any other specialty services you provide, like orthopedic surgery or hospice care, dental care, therapy laser, stem cell therapy, and all the specialty things that you do in addition to vaccines and annual or semi-annual exams. I think we'd all be surprised at the number of people that don't realize all we are capable of doing.

Part of this you can address in your monthly newsletters. You can talk about dental care. You can talk about preventative healthcare. You can talk about blood work and geriatric care and end-of-life care. You can highlight all those topics and that newsletter goes out to all your clients so you know they're aware of it. You can also design an infographic for your hospital or your clinic that talks about all the stages of life. If someone comes in with a new puppy, they'd be starting at the beginning of that spectrum. When you roll it out, you have middle-aged or older dogs, you would go over it with those clients, starting where their animal is at currently.

This would become something that you would lay out like a life plan, and you can start with puppyhood, first de-worming, first vaccines, clarify when you recommend starting heartworm prevention, when you start flea prevention, when do they get their last set of vaccines, at what age should they be spayed or neutered. Then moving on into adulthood, how often they need to have checkups, how often they need which vaccines, and any other specialty items, for example, when do we do dental exams? That's included in your annual exam. If we find something on that dental exam, then this is what we would do to address it. If we find a lump on a physical exam, this is what we'd do to address it. Go through all the possibilities on this educational page, which is basically map, a lifecycle of a client and the lifecycle of their pet. Go through all the possibilities, including at the end of life, what are your options. Will we come to your house and euthanize your pet? What are your options for caring for the body? Do you want to bury it in your backyard? Do you want to have it cremated? It'll lay out everything, so people, even if they have a puppy, they can look ahead and say, "Wow, there's a lot of things on here I didn't realize I needed to do for my pet or I didn't realize that you, as a veterinarian, could do for my pet."

It's going to open people's eyes. It's going to maximize your value to them and their visits to you, which will then maximize their value to you as as a client. It's a win-win situation. The client is going to get great healthcare for their animal, and you're going to get great business because of that, and because you've laid all this out. They now know that you do all of these things and what your recommendations are throughout life. Obviously, you're going to want to recommend the gold standard on this handout. What is ideal for your pet? If they approach you and say, "This is where we're at financially. We can't afford to do this part," then you can give them other options, but you want to know the best of the best is on this paper that you're handing out, on this lifecycle sheet.

This is one of the ways that you are going to maximize that lifetime value of your client and your patients. Many of the other things we've already talked about contribute to this as well. One of these is referrals. You want your clients to refer people who are like them to help your business and help themselves and their friend. We already talked about that being a win-win situation for both the referee and the referral. Another way to maximize their value is to make sure that all treatment plans are gone over thoroughly with your clients, so that they are followed through. If you offer laser therapy and they sign up for it, they need to know that they are going to be getting eight or nine sessions of laser.

Or if you offer physical therapy, what does that entail? What you want is to prepare them for what's coming, present that to them, have them accept your treatment plan and move forward.

You may need to have a specialized staff member that's trained in doing this, and that would be an amazing asset to your clinic and bottom line. Somebody that goes over estimates with clients for surgeries, for treatment plans, for anything that you're going to be doing with your patients because that person will have not only a good rapport with your clients, but they'll know how to explain these things so that the client sees the benefit in them for their pet. They will understand which is the best option, why they should do it, what's involved in doing it and then have the opportunity to commit to it. This team member will become great at explaining the details because they do it every day, all day.

This would also be a perfect place to introduce pet care plans if you offer those, either through your clinic or through one of the service providers, like Idexx or Partners for Healthy Pets. This is another way that you can maximize value and also get a commitment from your clients to your clinic. We underestimate the value of what people put on having a plan in place. They feel like it's almost an insurance policy for their pet, but it also commits them to coming back to *you* to follow through with that. This is another instance where it is a benefit for the client *and* a benefit for you. They have a monthly premium that they pay throughout the year. You know how much revenue's coming in from those plans each month and you get it paid up front. It evens out slow and busy months to some extent by having a predicable stream of income each month.

In Action

All these things that you do, both with your new clients and with your current clients to increase compliance are going to maximize the lifetime value of your customer and maximize your value to them. What we want is a happy, referring, healthy client and patient and we want our relationship with them to be a bond.

We want to provide the care to keep the animals healthy, as healthy as they can be, and that involves us providing great treatment options for them all the way through to end-of-life care. It also involves the client knowing what to expect at all steps along the way. We don't want to blindside them with something out of the blue, and that's were this client infographic, or client-patient lifecycle comes into play. It's not only going to benefit you and make your job easier because they have an idea what's coming, but it's going to benefit them because they can look ahead and plan for those things.

And all the special things you do to recognize your clients- the new client welcome package, the personalized cards, the events- are going to keep them coming back to you for all their needs.

For a template of a direct mail postcard designed to attract new clients, please visit www.vetclinicsuccesssecrets.com/mailer

Chapter 8. Customer Service Rules

"Do what you do so well that people can't help but tell others about you." - Walt Disney

The Game

Customer service rules. We've talked about all these different ways to keep you at the top of your clients minds. All the different promotions, how to get new clients walking in the door, but once they're there, you have got to make a great impression. If you don't, they're not going to stay. Your goal has got to be that once they come in your clinic, they never want to leave, because they feel welcome and know they can trust you. They are treated amazingly while they're there and you provide the services that they need.

So that's what we're going to talk about in this chapter, how to provide excellent and amazing customer service that keeps people talking and telling their friends about you.

The Plan

When people first walk in the door is your chance to make a first impression, a great first impression, so whoever mans the front is responsible for this. Your receptionist, and everyone who's up there, needs to turn around and greet clients warmly and with a smile as soon as they come in the door. If they know them by name, use their name in the greeting, we need to make them feel welcome from the moment that they walk in the door. If your receptionist is on the phone, she needs to look up and wave or smile and nod or somehow recognize the client who just entered. Your team needs to know that customers are not a distraction.

Your clients are the reason that they're there, and your clients are the ones who pay their paycheck. You may sign the check, but if you have no clients coming in the door paying for your services, there won't be money for them to get paid. So the first thing that all new employees should learn is the value of our clients and the importance of great customer service for them. You need to emphasize the importance of always greeting clients, and model this behavior. If you are talking with your receptionist when a client walks through the door, you also turn and greet them. If your high school cleaning kid is up front when a client walks in, teach them how to greet as well. Your whole clinic needs to be welcoming and friendly.

So it all starts the moment your client walks in the door. It also starts when you pick up the phone to answer any call that's coming in. It needs to be answered with a smile. You need to have a great greeting and it can be something super simple. "Good morning, this is Mountain Valley Veterinary Clinic. How may I help you today?" Everyone needs to have a smile on their face when they answer the phone, it makes a big difference. People can hear that. They can tell from across the phone lines that you are happy, you're ready to serve them, and what can they do for you? As long as there's a client in the office, they are number one, and the face to face client comes ahead of the phone call client. We still answer the phone. We still answer it pleasantly, but we don't sit and talk to them for 10 minutes while a client's standing in front of us, waiting.

Your receptionist should either ask them to hold and get someone else to help them, or finish with the client in front of them and then go back to the call. Ideally, if you have a couple people available, the second person can manage those phone calls coming in, even if you have two or three at the same time, while the first helps the client in the office. Those clients physically present need to know that they are a priority. With the client on the phone, you're going to train your staff to do what they can to help them out. They need to be trained to move them toward where they want to go. This means answering their question, scheduling an appointment, or taking a message. If they have a question or request the receptionist can't answer, there needs to be a policy in place of what to do next. I'm sure you've been on the receiving end of customer service frustration where you call somewhere and no one seems to be able to help you. Maybe it's with a problem. That seems to be when I experience this the most. I call a company and I have a problem. I have something that didn't happen right or something I need to return and I keep getting the "I'm sorry" lip service but really what I want is a solution, and you have to keep working your way up the line until you have to say, "Can I speak with your manager?" Oftentimes this is what it takes to get your solution.

That's not the way you want it to be in your practice. You want your staff to be able to deliver a solution to your clients. If that solution is talking to you, then that's probably not going to happen right at that moment. They can take a message if it's important, but most of the time, that solution is getting their animal an appointment. This enables you, as the vet, to figure out what's going on and solve the problem. This is going to be why the majority of clients are calling your office.

Another important thing to remember is that this attitude comes from the top down, so you have to value your clients and your patients and the staff has to know that. You have to model this behavior, so you can't be talking before your first appointment and say "Ugh, this woman's crazy. I can't stand her," and then walk in the room to see her and expect your staff to be on their best behavior with her afterwards. That is your leadership. You have to model the kind of behavior that you want from your staff. I think you'll find if you stop talking about any clients that way, your staff is going to pick up on that. They're going to treat them differently and you're going to notice a positive difference.

You also need to let your clients and your customers know that customer service is a priority for you, and if they have a problem, they need to tell you. You want them to talk to you so that the problem can be addressed and not overlooked, and not be something that you never know about or hear about. There are ways you can communicate this to your clients. One example would be a sign in the restroom that says, "Remember, the next person using this bathroom may be the one who determines the size of your next raise." Simple reminders like that, in places the public can see is a good thing. Not only will your clients realize your commitment to serving them, but your staff will read that when they are in the restroom, and leave it a little cleaner than they might have otherwise. You can even put in your newsletters, "Perfect customer service is our goal. If we don't meet your expectations, please let us know." Give a phone number where you can be reached. Something so people know that you are striving to provide an excellent experience.

In all reality, you shouldn't have to tell this to your clients. They should know it by the way you act when they come in the door. They should feel it coming from all of you, from the high school cleaners to the practice owners. If your cleaning people are mopping up front and someone walks in, their first job is to look up, smile and say "hello" to that person. We always want to make our clients feel welcome in our clinic, because they are the ones who pay for the clinic itself. They pay your salary, your staff's salary, and for all the equipment and the medicines that are used in the clinic.

This attitude of customer service is something that you have to revisit weekly. In every longer staff meeting, talk briefly, at least, about customer service. Maybe once a month you talk a little more in depth about it and how to deliver great customer service. Maybe you discuss an article you saw in the paper about great customer service, and also discuss examples of not-so-great customer service. One in the media recently that pops into mind is United Airlines forcible removal of a passenger. That was very, very poor customer service and it's going to be remembered for a long time. When you give great customer service, people feel good about themselves, they feel good about their decision to come in to your clinic, and they're going to tell their friends about it. But when they have a bad experience, they're probably going to tell even more people, so right there is a good reason to provide the best customer service possible. Besides, we want our clients to come back!

Part of providing good customer service is empowering your staff with answers, so they need to be well trained. They need to know the policies of the clinic, so when someone calls with a question, they can answer it. A big part of your team's customer service is going to be dealing with happy clients and normal clients. A smaller part of it is going to be dealing with unhappy clients, and they have to have the training to know how to deal with that too. We have a four letter acronym that we use for dealing with unhappy clients. It's called LEAR. L is for listen. Hear the client out, listen to their problem or complaint. E is for empathize. Try to understand where your client is coming from and what the true issue is. A is for Action. Take action to correct the problem, and R = resolve. Find a solution to the problem. That is the LEAR concept, you can have a cheat sheet by the phone stations to help your team remember this in the heat of the moment.

Your staff needs to see the problem from the clients point of view. They need to feel their pain, recognize the issue, and we say you have to get on the same level as the client. Because if they're mad about something and you're happy the whole time, they aren't going to like that. They're never going to feel like something has been resolved. You need to get down to their level, get frustrated alongside them and say, "Gosh, if I thought that was the case, I'd be frustrated too," or, "If something like that happened to me, I would be frustrated." You don't have to agree with what they're saying. You just have to validate their emotion, and that's an important thing to do if you're ever going to get them to come out of that anger mode. You have to meet them where they're at and bring them to where you want them to go, and that can be a tall order.

This is something that you need to work with your staff on so that they feel confident dealing with an unhappy client. Because truth be told, now most of the time someone calls and is mad or angry and yelling, they're going to put them on hold and come to you, wherever you are. If you want to avoid that in the future, although you are able to deal with it too, let your staff have the power and the confidence to deal with the situation. In order to do this, you need to give them some training so that they can understand what your goal is, which is to resolve the situation.

They need to understand where the person's coming from and bring them to a resolution that works for all of you.

One way that you can help them do this is give them not only the training but also some control, kind of an ace in their pocket. You can say, "You know what? If this situation arises, and no charging something or giving a refund for something, even though it's not typically our policy, if that is going to make this person happy or make them feel like you have heard their problem, you may." Then give them a dollar amount. Say, up to 50 dollars or whatever you want the limit to be, make that clear to them. This is something they can do without consulting with you first, they can use it when they need it. Most of the time they're not going to use this, but they know they've got it there, and that's going give them more confidence in dealing with an unhappy customer. You're also going to find that by doing this training, fewer clients are going to get to that unhappy place just because your staff is going to be better able to deal with them before a problem escalates.

They may be able to avert something by saying, "Gosh, you know, if that's really how you feel, let's not proceed today." Or maybe it will be something like "You're not happy with the charge for this, what if we split the cost with you? Because we did perform the procedure. We thought you wanted it. Turns out you don't. It was poor communication on our part. Here's what I can do to resolve that." They just validated the client's feelings, accepted partial responsibility, and offered a solution. The other thing you can do is ask the client "What can we do to make this right?" You might think you are opening a Pandora's box, but you'll be surprised at what people will ask for. Usually much less than you are anticipating. Very seldom will you get an unreasonable request. If you can talk to your staff, and let them know what the path of resolution looks like, and not to panic, they are going to be more confident and more willing to work with people who have a problem. They will learn to recognize when someone is heading towards having a problem, and that's going to be an invaluable tool for you as a manager because you're going be able to be less involved. You're empowering your staff so they feel more in control of their job and you're going to have less work in this area as well, which translates to fewer headaches and more time to do your job.

There are a lot of resources on customer relations that you can find. There are courses and books about this and other aspects of your training. You can find links at the end of this chapter as well.

There are a couple rules you should have for your staff about talking to your clients. One that we use is 'Never say anything to a client that you wouldn't say to your grandmother.' So, if you're going to say something, put grandma at the end of that, and if that still sounds okay to you, it's probably okay to say. A lot of times this is going to be when they're dealing with an angry client and tempted to say something that they may regret later or something that wouldn't reflect well on the clinic.

Sometimes it is not with angry or frustrated clients, but more common courtesy and politeness. Maybe someone's inquiring about certain procedures and your staff is tempted to say, "We don't do that here." Would you say, "We don't do that here, grandma?" Most people wouldn't say something that curt to grandma, and even though it's not a rude thing to say, you're not moving that client forward. If you are giving a client a negative answer, give them some ideas of what to do next. For example, "Well, we don't do that here, but maybe this specialty referral hospital does," or "Let me find out for you." Somehow you need to move them forward in what they're looking for, even if it's not you right now who can help them. At some point in the future, they're going to remember that you were helpful. And if they are calling you asking for something, chances are you're not the first place they've called, and they're still looking because no one helped them. No one moved them forward to where they wanted to go. This is one of the biggest ways you can improve your clients perception of your customer service, by helping them get where they want to go. When they call, they may not always know exactly what it is they need. But with proper questions and training, your staff will be able to help them discover what it is they are in need of. And to the client, this service is invaluable. It is going to make an impression, and they will appreciate you more for it.

Once the clients are in the clinic and in the exam room, and all the way through the checking out process, this impeccable service needs to continue. Respect your clients and their time. See them promptly in the exam room. If appointments are backing up, have someone tell them what to expect, and see what you can do to make them comfortable while they wait. Offer refreshments like bottled water or coffee for them, and even for the pet, too. If you keep them informed so they know what to expect and can plan for it, they will be much happier than if left in the dark about it. If you had an emergency come in the door that threw your schedule for a loop, let them know, and also offer to reschedule their appointment at another time if that would be more convenient. Or offer to have them leave the animal, and come back later if they would like. By keeping the lines of communication open, you are going to have happy clients. They will be much more willing to work with you if they know what is going on.

Great customer service also means doing what you say you'll do. If you say you'll call the client in 30 minutes about blood work results, do it. If your receptionist takes a message and says you'll call back shortly, it is her responsibility to make sure that happens. We need to give our clients reason to trust us and what we say. We all need to be a part of this incredible customer service, so our clients know we value them.

THE RESULT

When you emphasize the importance of customer service to your staff and present them with some initial training, you're going to hit a sore spot. We can all relate to poor customer service, because it seems that is becoming more and more the norm in our society. As you focus on providing great service, you will notice how poor the service is that you receive other places. You may stop frequenting restaurants because of this, and you'll bring stories back to your staff meetings. And this also gives you an advantage. You will stand out based on your customer service alone. Clients will be refreshed by your team's attitude and helpfulness. Your staff will start looking for other ways to exceed your client's expectations. You can even challenge them at a staff meeting: pose the question, "How can we improve our clients experience?" Have a sharpie and a big tablet and start writing. What of the things on this list can you implement right away? What needs some work and someone to be in charge of getting it ready to go? You will be surprised at how your staff can jump on this topic. And soon they will be bringing stories to you of their experiences with less than ideal customer service. And then you know you have them on board!

For more resources on customer service, please visit
www.vetclinicsuccesssecrets.com/customerservice

Chapter 9. The Huddle

"Do the difficult things while they are easy and do the great things while they are small. A journey of a thousand miles must begin with a single step." - Lao Tzu

Why Meet, Don't We All Work Here?

We had a staff meeting the other week, our once a week longer one, with a college girl scheduled to shadow for the day waiting in the lobby. By the time we went through our topics, did our stats, shared our 'wins', and went over the schedule, we were all laughing hard and joking and having fun. We were all on the same page, knew our numbers for the month, and were ready to face our day. When the college student joined us in the treatment area, she couldn't help but ask what had been so fun. Our laughter had filtered to the front of the clinic, and we were starting our day out on the right foot.

The Schedule

The morning meeting. One crucial thing that you need to do in your practice is have a meeting *every* morning, and this will be before the first scheduled appointment on the books. So if you start seeing appointments at nine am, this meeting needs to be at 8:45 or 8:30, preferably half an hour ahead of time to talk about what you need to and also to allow for any appointments that may be early. You don't want them interrupting you, and you do not want to make them wait.

At this meeting, you're going to talk about any hospitalized cases you have, almost like rounds. Go over any hospitalized animals, how they are this morning and how they did overnight. Your technicians or the kennel help should come prepared to give you the information you need on those animals, and then you have the opportunity to plan and then give your instructions for each case.

After addressing all the hospitalized patients, you move onto the schedule for the day. Have your receptionist print out what your schedule looks like, or if you do a handheld appointment book, bring that to the meeting so you can look down to the list and see what you have that day. Read each appointment out loud to give the staff a chance to fill you in on any details they may be aware of, and so the back office knows what's coming. If there are multiple doctors, everyone would be going over the whole schedule together. So if you're in charge, you read the whole schedule for each of the doctors as well as yourself. This way, you know what's coming in, what time they're coming, and have an idea of how the flow of your day is going to go. If you have surgeries first and then appointments, or appointments first and then a surgery you need to fit in, or any other procedures, you could figure out where to fit those into the schedule, or where they lie in the schedule as it is so you can plan accordingly.

After going over the schedule for the day, next on the agenda would be any unfinished business or items that need to be addressed. For example, any faxes from lab work or histopathology that had come in since the evening before, can be discussed. Any phone messages you or someone else needs to return or questions that have come in, that should be talked about as well. That way everybody is on the same page, everyone knows what's going on both with the schedule and with any follow-up that needs to be done. The technicians have their running instructions for the day for the hospitalized cases. Also address any surprises or any other issues that need to be talked about before the day begins. And lastly, go over the hospital numbers, where you are in both production and collections for the month.

This would be a time to bring up an emergency that called that is on its way in, and will give you a chance to figure out how you are going to work that into the schedule. Or if one of your receptionists got a call from an unhappy client, this would be when you bring it up. You talk about it, figure out what you're going to do, and take care of it.

This meeting may sound like a small thing, and really it is. It's easy to do, but it will make a huge impact on everyone in the hospital and also how smoothly your day flows. By knowing ahead of time what the game plan is, what the outline is, and realizing it may change a little bit during the day, you have a basic idea of what your day looks like. And so does the staff. So many times your team or the technicians in the back may not know what's going as far as appointments are concerned in the front of the hospital. And that communication between the back and the front is huge. You really need to have it in place to have a smooth running hospital where everybody knows what's going on, knows where their place is to help, what they need to be doing. It also improves the relations between the front and back of the hospital, which sometimes can be tenuous. If you have technicians in the back with no hospitalized patients and you don't have any surgeries that day, but you're booked solid with appointments, they can be up front cleaning rooms, and assisting in the exam rooms. It's nice for them to know that so they can plan what they need to do and where they need to be to help out.

You will be amazed at the change that this meeting gives your day, and the direction, and how it improves the flow of your day. In my practice, if we don't have that morning meeting, say, for example, because we have an emergency that comes in at 8:30, I am lost until we actually have a chance to sit down and talk about the schedule. And I know if you implement this, you'll find that, too. You'll find it is invaluable as far as your mental planning and how your day goes, just because you *know* what to expect. It's almost like scripting your day. You know what's coming in, what you need to deal with. And it also gives your mind and your subconscious a chance to think about the cases coming in, and differentials for them.

If you have a cat coming in and the person who took the appointment tells you what's going on with it, kind of weird signs, your mind's going to be working on that before you actually see that appointment, while you're doing all the things that happen before that. So by the time you get to that cat, you're going to have a few ideas about what you need to ask, what you need to do, or what may be going on with it.

This morning meeting is also a great time to talk about money, which is something that needs to be talked about in front of the whole staff. And a good thing to do is to track where you're at for both the year and the month, and to have a goal for each month. I know we've talked about this before, but you need to have set goals for each month, and for the year, so that you know where you're at, so the staff knows where you're at, and you all know what you need to do reach that goal. So, for example, every morning, you can say where production is this month, it's August fourth, and we are at $10,000. Where do you need to be for the month, how much do you have to go, all of that will give everybody an idea of what you need to be doing and where you're at.

So give both the production number and the collection number. If you have a large accounts receivable, this is a great place to address that. Because if you're talking about what the collections are for the month, say your production is $10,000 and your collections are $5,000, what's going on here? That gives you a chance to address that number before it becomes a giant monster by the end of the month. And if you do have a problem with collections, you probably know it already, and you may have a giant monster from the previous year that you're still dealing with. So this is a perfect time to show the staff some of these numbers so they know what you know, and can appreciate where your concern is coming from.

When you let somebody slide, "Oh yeah, you can pay on the first of the month," how is that affecting the bottom line? They'll see that every morning at this meeting and realize what the problem is, and where the money's going or not going. If you have implemented production-based bonuses, this is where they can show interest in tracking those numbers themselves. Once you get the employees onboard with those, they're going to be on top of it. They're going to know those numbers before you do. You'll show up to the meeting without them, and someone will say, "Hey, aren't we talking about numbers this morning?" And that's awesome, you want that! You want your employees to be tracking those numbers. Not because all you're concerned about is money, but because that's an essential part of running any business! You have to know where you're at money-wise. And you'll be amazed, by including in the employees in that, how it can influence the bottom line each month.

I think sometimes as business owners, we think that information isn't something for anyone else's eyes but our own. And while there's some validity to that statement, there's also huge value in sharing certain numbers with the staff so that they know where you're at and can plan for what they need to do to help the team reach the goals. Because it's not just your goals, they have to be clinic goals. You have to get everybody onboard if you're going to reach them.

So that is the morning meeting. Which needs to happen every day that you're going to be seeing appointments. And then once a week, it's a good idea to have a longer meeting where you can talk about other topics as well. Of course you always do the basics that we talked about for the morning meeting, but then at this longer meeting, you should add other topics. One of those things has to be stats. Once you have implemented a stat for all the positions, this is where they're going to show you their stats. They're will graph their numbers for each week, one month per sheet of graph paper, and at this meeting they're going to show those to you and to everybody else too. So everyone will see how each person's numbers look, and they're going to see where you're numbers are as well. Chances are, your stat is going to be your production. Each staff member will have their own number that differs depending on the stat for their position. But everyone has this graph they need to have completed and bring with them to share at the meeting.

One of the advantages of this is you can see in real time any trends. You will know the first week of the month versus the last week of the month, where everybody's numbers are, how they're doing, and where the business is headed. If everybody's stats are going down, that's a wake-up call. You've got to do something quickly about that. If one person's stats are down, but everybody else's are up, something's going on with that person or position and you need to address it. This gives you a chance to do so before it impacts everyone else and brings everyone else down too. So stats are one of the additional things you'll do at the longer meeting.

Another good idea is learning topics. Depending on what your staff needs to know, and this is a good opportunity to not segregate them into front and back office. Say you want to talk about lab tests. When we do lab work, some tests need to go in a serum separator tube, some go in a red top, and others in a lavender top or specialty tube. It's great for your receptionist to know what you're talking about when you say I need red top tubes. Or if she is calling the lab to find what is needed for a certain test, she knows what she needs to ask and what she's talking about. So if she has knowledge in this area, and others like it, everything will run more smoothly. Knowledge is power. And if you can help everybody learn, not to be an expert at someone else's job, but to know the basics, that's awesome. This was just one example of a simple topic, you may need to start there, or your staff may be way beyond that. It depends on how experienced they are. Don't overlook the new inexperienced one while trying to find new topics for the rest of the staff, or they will feel like they are not part of the team. Have one of the other staff members get up and teach a quick review of topics the new person needs to know. It will be a good review for one and great learning for the other.

Another good subject to talk about on these mornings is customer service. Remind everyone that your hospital goal is perfect customer service. Talk about any promotions that you have coming up, or any ideas for future promotions. Also do a learning session on anything that you want to do more of. So, say it's spring and you want to sell more heartworm prevention. Have a little morning session, 10 minute talk, on heartworm disease and why it is so important to be on prevention. Talk about why we test, why we recommend preventative, get everyone onboard. And then they're going to be asking every client that walks through the door, "Is your dog or your cat on heartworm preventative?" If they're not, they've got the power to say "Well let me tell you why we recommend it… Plus, we can do a heartworm test today and get you started on it!"

Now you have everyone involved, and your job just became easier. That client is pre-sold on the idea of heart worm prevention before you even walk in the room. So this is a good way to have special promotions of items that you want to do more of. Things that are going improve your bottom line as well as improve your patients' health. This is just a couple examples of things that you could do at these longer meetings. And you can have a schedule where you rotate through. For example, the first week of the month is customer service for your additional time. The second week, it is laboratory information, the third week, it's some type of service we're going provide more of. You can plan those things ahead of time, everybody will know what's coming, and it makes it easier on you every Thursday morning, or whenever you schedule this meeting, you're not going to be panicked the night before, trying to find something to talk about. You'll have it planned out ahead of time.

GOT IT

By implementing these morning meetings and the once a week longer staff meetings, you are going to notice a big change in your office as far as efficiency, productivity and communication. All of that is going to play together to your advantage. I know you'll find that like me, when you don't have this morning meeting, you'll be lost. You're going to wonder what's going on, what should be happening and what is scheduled later. By 10:30am you'll be saying "I can't take it! Everybody, come on, let's go meet, bring the schedule." So just try it, you'll love it!

For a sample list of topics of discussion and a meeting outline, visit www.vetclinicsuccesssecrets.com/meeting

Chapter 10. Business as Usual/ Communication

"Hard work opens doors and shows the world that you are serious about being one of those rare - and special - human beings who use the fullness of their talents to do their very best." - Robin S. Sharma

The Office

When you implement all of these things that we've talked about in the past nine chapters, in your clinic, you're going to be amazed at the results. You're going to see a higher productivity by great staff. They're going to be providing top of the line customer service to clients that you'll have coming in the door, due to your media and marketing and advertising, as well as your old clientele. You're going to be having more fun. You're going to be planning promotions, tracking your ads, having games that you can play with the staff to increase production, and all around have a smooth running, successful clinic.

Put It All Together

By implementing all the points we have discussed so far, you will see your practice change by leaps and bounds. It will become a place you love to show up at every day. You will enjoy the changes in attitude and service your rockstar employees are providing. They will be happy as well, taking pride in a job well done and being rewarded for it. You will have a better grasp on how to market your practice to attract new, ideal clients. All of you will be involved in planning fun new activities and events to position yourselves as the go-to place for veterinary care. Your clients will love you and send you their friends and associates. And they will feel valued in return, and know that you appreciate them. Every day you will be able to plan for what is coming your way, and your team will be prepared as well. You will have great communication throughout the clinic. Sound good? It can be!

By putting into place now the job descriptions and the hatting that we talked about, you'll be prepared for transition. Some of your current employees may leave as you implement this system, and that is just fine. You are sorting through to keep the good ones. If someone needs to leave, when you hire a new person, they can come in and pick up where that person left off. Granted, at first they won't be a pro, but you're going to have job descriptions that detail everything that that person is assigned to do, so they have the knowledge of what their job entails, what they're supposed to be doing and how to do it, and that gives them a feeling of control. They know what to expect, and they're going to perform better because of that. It will also give you a better idea sooner of their abilities and how they are going to work in the long run. Ideally, you'll discover this in the initial trial employment period.

The same is true for associate vets and relief vets, so that you can leave your practice in the hands of your staff, and someone else can come in and do your job for you. They're not going to be doing the marketing and the advertising and the management portion, unless you train them to do that, as you might with an associate, but they will be doing your job. and it should be easier because you have all these job descriptions written out of what *you* do, too. This enables you to take more time off, knowing that everything's going to be running smoothly while you're not there, and it's going to be fewer phones calls--hopefully, none!--to you, while you're on vacation. This is possible because your staff knows the policies, they know the routine, they're in control of their position, and there's not going to be much that they need to ask you about.

Implementing all of this will transition your practice into a turnkey operation. We think of practices now as being that when they're bought or sold, but that's really not the case. Rarely is there a training system, a manual of positions, with all these things in writing, all the procedures, that will make it a truly seamless and turnkey operation.

This is something you want to prepare for, even if you're not planning on your selling your practice right now. Maybe you just bought it a year or two ago, and you're trying to grow it, that's awesome! By you implementing these systems, your life is going to be smoother and easier, and when you are ready to transition out of or sell the practice, you're going to have those things in place. You're not going to be scrambling and working extra hard at that time, when you thought you could just be selling it, to get these systems in place.

Having all these systems also makes your practice more valuable to prospective buyers, and it makes it easier if you don't want to sell it, but you don't want to continue working either. You can have your staff and other veterinarians working, while you still maintain ownership of the practice, and everything will still run just as smoothly as it did while you were physically present. There are both short-term and long-term benefits to implementing these systems into your clinic.

The key to implementing all of this is going to be communication. You have to have open and good communication lines between you and your staff, especially your staff, and anyone else that comes in to work, like a relief vet or an associate vet. You must have procedures in place to allow that communication.

For example, when you bring a new team member on board, you need to schedule upfront personal development interviews, so that you and they know what to expect and when you're going to talk about it. Overall these personal development interviews should be upbeat. You should go over all the things that they're doing great, what things they can improve upon in their job to make them even more valuable to you, to raise their stats, to make them feel that they have more control and ownership of their position. This also gives you a set time to review everything, versus "when I have time." The more things are spelled out and scheduled ahead of time, the fewer surprises you're going to run into, and, I don't know about you, but surprises in business are rarely a good thing.

This open communication is going to take some time and some effort on your part. You're going to have to talk to your staff about what you expect. In chapter 4, we reviewed that some of your staff may not make this transition with you, and that's completely okay. You're better off without them. The ones that do, need to know that this is the new policy. This is how we're going to communicate and have it spelled out, so nobody has any questions. If they do, you address those, and you add those to your procedures manual, so that you don't have to address it individually in the future. It will already be spelled out.

The same is true with any other procedures or job descriptions. If a question comes up, address it. If there's a better way to do it, fix it, and then update your manual, update those positions, so that you aren't doing the same thing over and over again. You want everyone to be as efficient as possible, and pre-emotively answer any questions that may arise.

I think that happens to a lot of us now. If you don't have these in place, and you hire a new technician, you're going through the exact same things with her or him that you did with the previous one you hired. That's one of the things that wears us out and burns us out, as far as the employee management side. Who wants to beat their head against a wall for training purposes? When, if it was all spelled out, we're not answering that same question, over the course of a year, 25 times? We're answering it once, writing it out once, and then, if there's a question, that person can go and look it up in their job description.

It's going to make your life easier, because you won't be dealing with the repetition portion of that. It's going to give you fewer headaches. The staff will be happier, because, a lot of times, they don't want to come to you or to their superior and ask a question. You want them to be *able* to do that, but you also want someone that's going to take the initiative and say, "I know this answer is somewhere. I'm going to look it up in my job description."

That person, and that type of person, is someone who likes to control their own destiny, and that's what you want. You want someone who takes ownership of their position and who works to improve that position. Like we just talked about, if there's something that they think can be done better a different way, open those lines of communication. Tell them, "If that's the case, then write out your better solution. Come to me. Let's review both and update it if we need to," so that it does work better in the future.

It might seem like a lot of work to you now, but it *is* going to pay off. You'll have fewer interruptions, fewer distractions. You'll be able to focus on your job a greater percentage of the time, instead of on the management portion, and specifically, the employee management portion. Your highest productive activity is either practicing veterinary medicine or doing the advertising and marketing that's going to get your clients back in the office and new clients walking through the door. That's where you can be the greatest asset. You don't want to be spending 50% of your time managing your employees and doing the same things over and over again, as far as training or policy review goes, when you could be doing these higher productive activities.

Back to the staff and opening these lines of communication. In one of your staff meetings, you need to talk about communication and define it, really. One of the management companies that we have worked with has some great definitions for communication and also relationships, and I'm going to go over a couple of those.

With communication, it's a two-way street. You need to have the intent to communicate with someone else. They need to have attention to receive that communication, and that involves both words and body language. You need to be looking at someone, making eye contact, and open to what they are saying. When you're teaching your staff about these new procedures and about how to deal with unhappy clients, they need to be paying attention. There has to be intention and attention, so that the communication is understood by both parties. When it is, you should know it. Your team should be able to repeat back to you exactly what you're talking about and understand it. If they don't, that's a perfect time to ask questions.

This also needs to be applied, by you and your staff, towards clients. We need to be looking at them when we're talking to them. When we ask a question, we need to be ready to receive that answer and understand it, so that we have an open line of communication. Most problems in practice, as far as clients go, are related to a lack of communication, and it's something I think we, as veterinarians, don't always do as well as we should. It's not something we're taught in school. There was no class on communication or client relations, or at least there wasn't when I went to school. This is an area where both you and your staff can work together and with clients to improve this.

There is a communication tool, called the ARC triangle, that will help you in this. The A stands for affinity; R stands for reality; C stands for communication. With this triangle, as with a solid triangle, if you imagine a metal dinner bell, the kind that used to hang outside old ranch houses, you can't raise just one corner of it without raising the whole thing. If you can raise any portion of that triangle with your clients or with your staff, the whole relationship is going to move to another level. You will reach a new level of understanding.

Let's take affinity, for example ... Affinity is liking or wanting to be near something or someone, or disliking or not wanting to be near. If you can increase your affinity with someone, your relationship is going to step up a level. One way to increase the affinity is by increasing your shared reality. Say you have a client in the waiting room, and she's wearing a beautiful red dress. Compliment her on that, say "Wow, that's a beautiful red dress you're wearing." You are acknowledging the reality of a red dress. You are complimenting her on it, because it is a pretty dress. It must be a sincere compliment, too, no empty flattery, but you're recognizing her reality, and thus sharing that reality. You're increasing her affinity toward you, because everyone likes to be complimented, which is going to enable your communication to increase as well. You're going to have a higher rate of customer or client compliance when you have them liking you, having a higher affinity toward you and a closer reality. This raises that whole triangle up. You can also approach this from the reality of their pet. It may seem obvious, but say something like, "What a white Shih Tzu you have. She sure is a pretty girl." You are acknowledging the reality of the color, breed and gender of the dog, which immediately expands your shared reality. The owner realizes you are paying attention, and immediately is more open to your communications.

This is something fun to practice with people, with your staff and with your clients. It's interesting to watch how your staff will respond to this, too. Once they learn these techniques, they're going to be using them, because they are so helpful. They're going to be practicing them, not only at your clinic, but when they go out to dinner. They're going to say something to the waitress that's going to increase their shared reality or increase their affinity for one another, and they're going to receive better service. You know you've made an impression when they come to your morning meeting and tell you the story of how they used the ARC triangle at dinner last night. I learned this technique from one of the consulting companies we have hired, and it is worth its weight in gold. This is just a brief description, but as always, more information can be found at the link at the end of this chapter.

As I just mentioned, this plays into all parts of life, but your primary focus is how it makes your office run more smoothly. Your whole team understands what's involved in the client relationship and the communication. When you put it to work, everything is going to go a lot more smoothly. You'll notice everyone is going to be happier, too. Everyone will be more upbeat. When you enjoy what you're doing, and you have control of your life, just like we talked about with the employees ... When they have control of their position, and they have ownership of it, it leads to a more satisfied outlook and content personality. That will be shared throughout the office, and that itself is a beautiful thing.

In conclusion, when you implement all of these things in your practice, you're going to notice an amazing difference. Imagine for a moment what that will look like in your clinic. Stop reading, close your eyes and picture the happy staff, all doing their jobs, just the way you designed. The clients coming in, leaving compliant and very pleased with the service and the results. Your job pleasant and enjoyable, like you envisioned it would be when you graduated from vet school. A turnkey operation that will be ready to sell whenever you are ready, and so much more valuable to you in the meantime than a 'fly by the seat of your pants' clinic. You will never regret the effort you put into doing this. It will take a little bit of ongoing maintenance, like we talked about. The opportunity for that will be at the weekly meetings, you need to talk about customer service and statistics and go over all those things in turn. Direct your energy to what you want to improve. What you focus on expands.

If you're tracking everyone's production, it's going to improve. If you're tracking your clinic's numbers, those are going to improve. If you're tracking the number of new clients that you have, that's going to improve as well. All of this is basic management of your clinic, designed specifically for us, as veterinarians, so that we can do the part of practice that we love and not spend as much time on the part that we don't enjoy. If you enjoy the management part, great. This will be a fun challenge for you. If, at the moment, it's not your favorite part, go through these exercises. I think you'll find that you don't dread the employee management part as much as you did before you read this book and implemented these techniques. You may find, like me, that this becomes your favorite part of clinic life!

Work is going to become more fun. You're going to have an improved staff, and that alone will make it more enjoyable. This is the ounce of prevention that's worth more than a pound of cure. By putting in the effort now, you're going to benefit a month down the road, six months down the road, and 10 years down the road. You're going to make your life easier, more fun, and your clinic more fun and a place that you want to be. It's going to be a place your employees want to be, demonstrated by long-lasting careers and great production. It's all going to come together to make your life better, both practice success wise and personal success wise. You'll find that when you're not stressed out over the management portion or not having any new clients come in or not being able to pay the bills, that personal stress is going to melt away, too. You'll be happier at home, at work and in life in general. Life is too short to waste being unhappy. Live your dream now!

The Long Haul

There will be times you may get off-course. You may drift back to previous work habits and the team may slack a little on customer service. This happens. I believe it is called the Chaos Theory ;). Just learn to recognize it and get back on track. It's okay, move forward, go easy on yourself. This whole practice ownership thing is hard work!

Congratulations on looking for a better way, and reaching out, reading this book.

The tools here will allow your whole practice to come together like cogs in a wheel. It will be a seamless interaction between your patients, your clients, your staff, yourself, your marketing. All of it will work together to drive this machine called the veterinary clinic. When things get tough, remember your dream practice. Take a few deep breaths and go over the basics. What can you do now to move things in the direction you want?

As always, I am in this for your success. If there's anything else that I can provide or ways I can be of service to you, don't hesitate to reach out. There are a lot of resources available to you. I want you to succeed. I want you to enjoy your life. I want your practice to be successful and to be exactly where you want it to be.

For more in depth instruction on how to get your practice up to speed, and learn about the ARC triangle, visit www.vetclinicsuccesssecrets.com/makeitwork

About The Author

SUSIE HIRSCH, DVM Susie is a 20 year veteran of the world of vet med. A practice owner since 1999, she has been through the ups and downs of practice ownership, employee management, and cycles of the economy.

Susie raises registered Pinzgauer cattle, and derives great satisfaction from the agricultural side of her life. She has raised yaks for several years as well, but recently sold the yak herd to get into reindeer.

Susie has homeschooled her children at the vet clinic, although currently all but one are in public school.

She is also active in her church and coaches youth soccer.

Susie's mission now is to use her experience to help other veterinarians who are struggling with practice ownership and success. She is still working in her clinic, but cutting back to pursue more of the management and marketing side.

Susie lives in western Colorado with her husband Jeff and their four children, and a farm full of animals.

Connect with Susie elsewhere:

Facebook: https://www.facebook.com/DrSusieHirsch
Google+:
LinkedIn: https://www.LinkedIn.com/in/SusieHirsch

Amazon Author Page: amazon.com/author/susiehirsch

OTHER OFFERINGS FROM SUSIE

Susie has a couple other products that will help veterinarians. The first is "The Client Delivery System," which is a quick action plan on how to get more new clients into your clinic next month, including everything you need to get it done now. The second is a four week webinar-based course that offers more in-depth information and tools for your practice success. Offering many templates and done-for-you examples, it is the fast track to implementing this organization in your clinic. A monthly newsletter with ready-to-use marketing items accompanies the course, and helps keep you on the path to success.
Visit www.vetclinicsuccesssecrets.com/course for more information.

ONE LAST THING...

If you enjoyed this book or found it useful I'd be very grateful if you'd post a short review on Amazon. Your support really does make a difference and I read all the reviews personally so I can get your feedback and make this book even better.

If you'd like to leave a review then all you need to do is click the review link on this book's page on Amazon here:

https://www.amazon.com/dp/B071GQK1R8/ref=cm_cr_ryp_prd_ttl_sol_0

Thanks again for your support!

www.ingramcontent.com/pod-product-compliance
Lightning Source LLC
Chambersburg PA
CBHW020929180526
45163CB00007B/2938